T0301776

Regenerative Medicine, Artificial Cells
and Nanomedicine – Vol. 2

Present and Future Therapies
for End-Stage Renal Disease

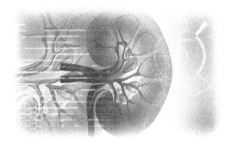

Regenerative Medicine, Artificial Cells and Nanomedicine – Vol. 2

Present and Future Therapies for End-Stage Renal Disease

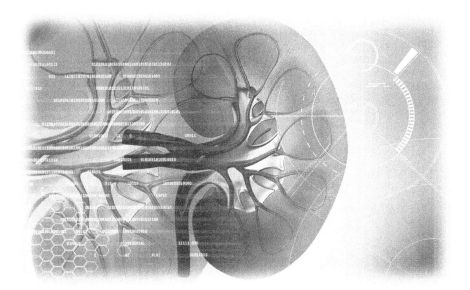

Editors

Eli A Friedman
Mary C Mallappallil

SUNY Downstate Medical Center, USA

World Scientific

NEW JERSEY · LONDON · SINGAPORE · BEIJING · SHANGHAI · HONG KONG · TAIPEI · CHENNAI

Published by

World Scientific Publishing Co. Pte. Ltd.

5 Toh Tuck Link, Singapore 596224

USA office: 27 Warren Street, Suite 401-402, Hackensack, NJ 07601

UK office: 57 Shelton Street, Covent Garden, London WC2H 9HE

Library of Congress Cataloging-in-Publication Data
Present and future therapies for end-stage renal disease / editors, Eli A. Friedman,
Mary C. Mallappallil.
    p. ; cm. -- (Regenerative medicine, artificial cells and nanomedicine ; v. 2)
    Includes bibliographical references and index.
    ISBN-13: 978-9814280020 (hardcover : alk. paper)
    ISBN-10: 981428002X (hardcover : alk. paper)
    1. Chronic renal failurexTreatment. 2. Hemodialysis. I. Friedman, Eli A., 1933–
II. Mallappallil, Mary C. III. Series: Regenerative medicine, artificial cells and
nanomedicine ; v. 2.
    [DNLM: 1. Kidney Failure, Chronic--therapy. 2. Renal Dialysis--methods.
3. Kidney Transplantation. WJ 378 P933 2010]
    RC918.R4P677 2010
    616.6'14--dc22

                                                                    2010000016

British Library Cataloguing-in-Publication Data
A catalogue record for this book is available from the British Library.

Copyright © 2010 by World Scientific Publishing Co. Pte. Ltd.

*All rights reserved. This book, or parts thereof, may not be reproduced in any form or by any means,
electronic or mechanical, including photocopying, recording or any information storage and retrieval
system now known or to be invented, without written permission from the Publisher.*

For photocopying of material in this volume, please pay a copying fee through the Copyright Clearance
Center, Inc., 222 Rosewood Drive, Danvers, MA 01923, USA. In this case permission to photocopy
is not required from the publisher.

Typeset by Stallion Press
Email: enquiries@stallionpress.com

Printed in Singapore

Contents

Introduction and Options in Therapy

*Eli A. Friedman**

At the close of 2009, as this is revised, the severity and course of progressive chronic kidney disease (CKD) is defined by the National Kidney Foundation Kidney Disease Outcomes Quality Initiative[1] in five stages, with diagnostic and management guidelines for each. Based upon estimated GFR (eGFR) values calculated from serum creatinine measurements, along with determination of urine albumin concentration, the stages are (see Table 1):

- Stage 1 CKD is present when there is evidence of kidney damage with a normal eGFR.
- Stage 2 CKD is present when there is kidney damage and decrease in the eGFR to 60–89 ml/min. Stage 1 or 2 CKD may be diagnosed through hypertension, hematuria or proteinuria, or a family history of kidney disease such as polycystic kidney disease. Supernormal levels of creatinine and/or urea in the blood are common.
- Stage 3 CKD is diagnosed by a reduced eGFR of 30–59 ml/min. Anemia and early metabolic bone disease may be detected.
- Stage 4 CKD is present when the eGFR falls to 15–29 ml/min. Most patients complain of fatigue, loss of appetite, difficulty in sleeping at night, reduced concentrating ability, and a loss of sexual drive.
- Stage 5 CKD is present when the eGFR falls below 15 ml/min.

*Distinguished Teaching Professor of Medicine, Downstate Medical Center, 450 Clarkson Avenue, Brooklyn, New York, 11203, USA. Email: Elifriedman@aol.com

Table 1.   Stages of Chronic Kidney Disease

Stage	Description	eGFR[a] (mL/min/1.73 m^2)
1	Slight kidney damage with normal or increased filtration	More than 90
2	Mild decrease in kidney function	60–89
3	Moderate decrease in kidney function	30–59
4	Severe decrease in kidney function	15–29
5	Kidney failure requiring dialysis or transplantation	Less than 15

[a]Estimated glomerular filtration rate — a measurement of the kidney function calculated from serum creatinine concentration.

Interpreted by George E. Schreiner, the evolution of the medical–industrial complex that provides contemporary therapy for stage 5 CKD is the result of "so few stimulating so many!"[2] The story began when Willem J. Kolff (who died in February 2009 at the age of 97), stimulated modern therapy for acute kidney failure by both application of peritoneal dialysis and fabrication of a workable artificial kidney in 1943 under the German occupation of The Netherlands.[3]

In Boston, after his return from World War II service, John P. Merrill's Peter Bent Brigham Hospital Team redesigned Kolff's artificial kidney, affirming its utility in short-term substitution for failed kidneys.[4] Subsequently, the team's kidney transplantation in monozygotic twins initiated transplant medicine as a discipline.[5] Concurrently, Schreiner at Georgetown Hospital in Washington D.C., one of the 13 founders of the American Society of Nephrology and the "handful" of people who created the American Society for Artificial Internal Organs (ASAIO), pointed out that it was the increasing success in sustaining patients of acute renal failure for six or more months that stimulated the quest for long-term uremia therapy. After Belding H. Scribner, in 1960, reported his Seattle team's ongoing life prolongation in two uremic patients by "chronic hemodialysis" via an external Teflon radial arteriovenous shunt,[6] it became starkly evident that biotechnology could substitute for loss of a vital organ system.

When Scribner showed how dialysis could pre-empt death in stage 5 CKD, nephrology did not exist as either a discipline or a specialty, though groups of investigators and clinicians around the world maintained interest in kidney function, pathology, and clinical diseases. The International Society of Nephrology (ISN), at its first meeting in Evian, France, in 1960, attracted fewer than 100 attendees. Following Scribner's impact, however, at the American Society of Nephrology's (ASN) 1966 initial meeting, held jointly with the ISN, in Washington D.C., attendance reached 3000, signaling that nephrology was here to stay. Reaction to Scribner's report in the *ASAIO Transactions* combined surprise, disbelief, and excitement. The Public Health Service rapidly funded several "demonstration centers" to authenticate the validity of the Seattle "accomplishment" and formed an expert committee to explore funding mechanisms for advancing chronic hemodialysis as a treatment available throughout America.

For undecipherable reasons, the United States Congress, after reviewing the growing number of strongly positive reports from hemodialysis demonstration projects established by the Chronic Disease Division of the Public Health Service, in 1972, selected the term "end-stage renal disease" (ESRD) for what is currently called stage 5 CKD. Collaboration between the National Kidney Foundation, the ASN, and patient activist groups was able to convince the Ways and Means Committee of Congress to amend the Social Security Act (Public Law 92-603) to extend coverage for ESRD under Medicare. Indeed, individuals eligible for Medicare because of ESRD became entitled to all benefits available under the Medicare program, not just ESRD-related dialysis and kidney transplantation. Despite appreciation of the reality that no person wants to be considered an end-stage failure in anything, the designation has persisted until today. Further amendments in 1978 (Public Law 95-292) revised Medicare rules to encourage self-dialysis and kidney transplantation.

To gain ESRD benefits, a physician must certify that the individual requires chronic dialysis or a kidney transplant to maintain life. In addition to having chronic renal failure, the person must either be entitled to a monthly insurance benefit under title 11 of the Social Security Act (or an annuity under the Railroad Retirement Act), be fully or currently insured under Social Security (railroad work may count), or be the spouse or dependent child of a person who meets one of the previous requirements.

Medicare ESRD entitlement begins when whichever of the following is earliest:

- The third month after the month in which dialysis is initiated.
- The month in which dialysis begins if the individual participates in self-dialysis training at an approved facility and is expected to self-dialyze thereafter.
- The month of a kidney transplant.
- The month of admission to an approved hospital for procedures preliminary to a transplant, if the transplant takes place within the following two months. If the transplant is delayed by more than two months, coverage starts in the second month prior to the month in which the transplant takes place.

Medicare ESRD coverage terminates when whichever of the following is earliest:

- The day of death.
- The last day of the 12th month after ending maintenance dialysis treatments.
- The last day of the 36th month after a kidney transplant. Re-transplantation within 36 months or return to dialysis does not interrupt the entitlement.

A person whose ESRD entitlement terminates continues with the entitlement if disabled or 65 years or older.

Nephrology began as a medical specialty once it became possible to forestall death from kidney failure by the use of devices and regimens that could be passed from teacher to student. It was also true that nephrology spurred a rebirth of medical ethics as there was recognition of the limitations on delivering ESRD treatments imposed by economics and other variables enumerated in Table 2.[7]

Table 2.   Ethical Stresses Induced by Ability to Extend Life in ESRD

1. Is indeterminate life extension using a machine moral?
2. Must a physician propose machine-facilitated life extension to patients at the end of life?
3. What criteria should be used to begin ESRD therapy?
   a. An arbitrary eGFR below 10 ml/min?
   b. A nephrologist's clinical judgment that treatment is indicated?
   c. The patient's request irrespective of the eGFR?
   d. A family member or legal representative's request?
4. Does society (the government) have the right or obligation to regulate life extension?
5. Should a mentally incompetent person receive life extension by dialysis if he or she:
   a. Is demented?
   b. Is psychotic?
   c. Has a low IQ?
   d. Has respiratory intubation?
6. If demand for dialysis life extension exceeds supply, should allocation be decided by:
   a. Government?
   b. Physician?
   c. Committee (hospital or community)?
   d. Ethicist?
   e. Clergy?
7. When allocating scarce resources such as deceased-donor kidneys, should priority be determined by:
   a. Individual ability to pay?
   b. Social merit?
   c. Citizenship?
   d. Race?
   e. Gender?
   f. Age?
   g. Marital status?
   h. Employment status?
8. Should government remuneration to physicians permit:
   a. Corporate ownership (for profit) of dialysis units?
   b. Physician ownership of dialysis facilities?
   c. Self-referral of dialysis patients?

(Continued)

Table 2.   *(Continued)*

9. Must dialysis-based life extension at government expense be proscribed for:
    a. Criminals incarcerated for serious crimes (murder, rape)?
    b. Recidivist substance abusers (narcotics, alcohol)?
    c. Persistently nonadherent patients (smokers, morbidly obese)?
    d. Transplant tourists who purchased marketed organs (kidneys)?
    e. Incarcerated terrorists who have injured innocent civilians?
    f. HIV + persons?

Consider the extent of decisions that might be prompted by the next uremic patient entering a modern emergency room with newly recognized advanced renal failure. After life-threatening hyperkalemia, pericardial tamponade, and bleeding are managed by urgent dialysis, if appropriate, assessment of the patient must address at least some of the following issues: (1) Which form of dialysis (peritoneal dialysis or hemodialysis) should be considered for the long term? (2) Is self-care or home dialysis the preferred option? (3) How can the patient be prepared for an informed decision as to whether or not to undergo kidney transplantation? (4) For this specific patient, is a live-donor or deceased-donor kidney preferable? The list goes on, underscoring the rationale for the topics of chapters included in this text.

No universal correct answers to the complex questions posed in Table 2 may be given without reflection on a specific patient's circumstances. It is the intent of this text to ease the burden of decision by discussing the major ESRD therapies in light of who might be best for which, when. Not addressed in Table 2, however, is the sad reality that the cost of uremia therapy is beyond the majority of the world's population.[8] Neither China nor India, as examples of nations with a population of greater than 1 billion, is able to treat even 5% of its ESRD patients. Similarly, for Sierre Leone, The Congo, Chad, North Korea or Uruguay, desperate concerns over feeding people defeat any effort to construct an ESRD program. Thus, consideration of one hope for the future — administration of probiotic bacteria deploying the gut as a substitute kidney — is included as a chapter, mainly to remove limitation in thinking about how kidney failure may be treated in the near future. Willem J. Kolff, who died in 2009 at 97, did not, as he performed the first hemodialysis using sausage casing and heparin, 55 years earlier, imagine a world in which more than 1 million people would be alive because he discerned a means of stopping otherwise inevitable deaths due to the loss of kidney function.

References

1. KDOQI. (2007) KDOQI clinical practice guidelines and clinical practice recommendations for diabetes and chronic kidney disease. *Am J Kidney Dis* **49**(Suppl 2): S12–S154.
2. Schreiner GE. (2000) How end-stage renal disease (ESRD) Medicare developed. *Am J Kidney Dis* **35**(Suppl 1): A37–S44.
3. Kolff WJ. (1947) *New Ways of Treating Uraemia: Artificial Kidney, Peritoneal Lavage, Intestinal Lavage.* J & A Churchill, London.
4. Merrill JP, Smith S III, Callahan EJ III, Thorn GW. (1950) The use of an artificial kidney. II. Clinical experience. *J Clin Invest* **29**: 425–438.
5. Merrill JP, Murray JE, Harrison JH, Guild W. (1956) Successful homo-transplantations of the human kidney between identical twins. *JAMA* **160**: 277–282.
6. Scribner BH, Buri R, Caner JEZ, *et al.* (1960) The treatment of chronic uremia by means of intermittent dialysis. *Trans Am Soc Artif Intern Organs* **6**: 114–121.
7. Friedman EA. (1998) Kolff's contributions provoked the birth of ethics in nephrology. *Artif Organs* **13**: 46–51.
8. Friedman EA. (2003) Restating the obvious: the world can't afford American health care (*editorial*). *ASAIO J* **49**: 507–509.

PART 1

Contemporary Uremia Therapy CIRCA 2009

CHAPTER 1

Peritoneal Dialysis: Past and Current Practices

Mary C. Mallappallil*

History of Peritoneal Dialysis

The peritoneal membrane was first described by ancient Egyptians. In 1923, Georg Ganter at the University or Wurzburg in Germany infused one liter of a specially prepared solution into the abdomen of a patient with obstructive uropathy, which temporarily helped the patient, who eventually died.[1] In 1938, Jonathan Rhoads added lactate to the peritoneal dialysate solution to combat acidosis. Even though sterilized material was used, safe and repeated access to the peritoneum was limited. Many investigators attempted to improve the technology used for peritoneal dialysis, including Arthur Grollman, who in 1952 at the Southwestern Medical School in Dallas tried to use a one-liter dialysate container with a plastic tube and a cap. Paul Doolan, in 1959, devised a catheter that would clog less frequently. Finally, in 1968, Henry Tenckhoff devised the currently employed catheter made of silicone with two cuffs that allowed the catheter to stay in place between treatments, rather than the previous method which required a new catheter placement at each treatment session.

---

*Assistant Professor of Medicine, Downstate Medical Center, 450 Clarkson Avenue, Brooklyn, New York, 11203, USA.

Landmarks in Technologies and Techniques in the Last Half-Century

Plastic bags

Once repeat access to the peritoneum was possible, peritoneal dialysis was still limited by the frequent occurrence of peritonitis. Through 1978, commercially marketed dialysate solution was available only in glass containers that were connected to the catheter with plastic tubing. Attributed to the multiple connections, the frequency of peritonitis prevented the expansion of peritoneal dialysis as a broadly utilized option for uremia therapy. Oreopoulos, in Toronto, Canada, introduced peritoneal dialysate solution in plastic bags that needed fewer connections. The first connection allowed the fluid to flow into the peritoneum and, after dwelling for an assigned time, the fluid drained back into the bag by gravity, after which a new bag could be connected. With plastic bags and fewer connections a decrease in the incidence of peritonitis followed.

Y system

The Y system, devised in Italy by Umberto Buoncristiani, decreased the number of peritonitis episodes in comparison with the then standard flow pattern in 1983.[2] The catheter and the tail of the Y were closed while the tubing was flushed with fresh solution. Only after the tubing was flushed was the abdominal catheter opened, and unspent dialysate was allowed into the peritoneum. The Y system with the flush before use further decreased the incidence of peritonitis, from one episode of peritonitis every 11 patient months to one every 33 patient months.[3]

Double bag system

In 1991, a commercially introduced double bag system based on the Y principle with an empty bag and one with solution further reduced the number of disconnects and connections. The patient was required to make only one connection with a disposable system, resulting in a 63% probability of peritonitis-free patients at 24 months.[4]

Continuous ambulatory peritoneal dialysis

In 1975, Popovich and Moncrief started what they called continuous ambulatory peritoneal dialysis (CAPD) in a patient unable to tolerate hemodialysis. After evaluating CAPD in 9 patients over 136 patient weeks, they concluded that if infection could be reduced, CAPD was an attractive option for uremia therapy.[5] The steady flow and deposit of fluid into the peritoneal cavity allowed more stable removal of solutes and fluids when compared to intermittent therapies.

Automated peritoneal dialysis

Boen at Washington University developed an automated cycling machine that held large amounts of peritoneal dialysate solution.[6] This technology was refined by Tenckhoff to allow concentration and an easier manipulation of the solution.

Compact cycler machine

In the 1990s, the use of an automated cycler in what was termed continuous cyclic peritoneal dialysis (CCPD) extended the options for uremia therapy available to patients.

Dialysate solutions

A perfect solution would remove waste including water while supplementing essential nutrients with no absorption of unnecessary compounds. In reality, most dialysate solutions are used based on their side effect profiles. The osmotic component of peritoneal dialysate is carbohydrate and absorbable sugars, which are detrimental because of the formation of advanced glycosylation end products (AGEs) resulting in damage to the peritoneal membrane over time.

A less absorbed glucose polymer, icodextran, which is absorbed at a lower rate than glucose, is now increasingly being used to limit AGE formation.

Amino acid solutions have also been employed in an attempt to minimize protein loss during peritoneal dialysis, with inconsistent results. Early trials did not improve the nutritional status, while a study by Kopple *et al.* showed some benefit, in terms of net protein intake, and noted an increase in acidosis and a rise in blood urea nitrogen levels.[7]

Removal of the high clearance target

Both the ADMEX and Hong Kong trials in 2002 and 2003 respectively prompted the NKF/K DOQI 2006 guidelines to reduce the previously targeted minimal Kt/V from >2 to 1.7 by taking into account residual renal function.[8,9]

Epidemiology

According to the United States Renal Data System report, there were 26,114 prevalent peritoneal dialysis patients as of December 31, 2006, including continuous and automated peritoneal dialysis. Concurrently, the number of prevalent patients on hemodialysis was 327,754, while those with a functioning kidney transplant numbered 151,502.[10] Worldwide there are about 150,000 patients with end stage renal disease on peritoneal dialysis.

Several studies have compared peritoneal dialysis to in-center hemodialysis and found no advantage in one versus the other modality in the long term. At initiation of renal replacement therapy a slight survival advantage was noted in peritoneal dialysis, attributed to patient selection of younger, more functional patients which was not present after the period of one year.[11] A prospective comparison of mortality was done by Jaar *et al.* in a seven-year cohort study of 1041 patients from 81 hemodialysis and 19 peritoneal centers in the USA. The authors noted that 25% of patients on peritoneal dialysis were likely to change modality and 5% in the hemodialysis group.

Mortality did not differ in the two groups in the first year, after which period the mortality was shown to increase in the peritoneal dialysis group.[12]

Disappearance of peritoneal dialysis has been noted in the USA among incident end stage kidney disease patients despite improvement in techniques and outcomes from 11% in 1996 to 7% in 2003.[13] In 1991, Kimmel *et al.* noted a lack of satisfaction among trainees in nephrology fellowship regarding peritoneal dialysis.[14]

While most developed nations have more hemodialysis than peritoneal dialysis, an exception is Australia, where peritoneal dialysis is the first choice of renal replacement therapy. Two important factors are at work here: in Australia Aboriginal people have more end stage renal disease than the rest of the population, and these patients live in distant areas covered by the Remote Area Health Services, which may be thousands of kilometers from dialysis centers.[15,16]

Typical Use

The placement of dialysate into the peritoneum allows the clearance of nitrogenous waste and electrolytes along with ultrafiltration of excess fluid. The force driving ultrafiltration has been the concentration of glucose in the dialysate, prompting, until recently, concern over the caloric content absorbed leading to the formation of AGEs and the eventual loss of the membrane. The slower shift of materials is more physiologic when compared to three-times-a-week in-center hemodialysis. While an inadequate dialysis dose has been a concern in large patients, the concept is mainly unproven and the size of any patient should not exclude him or her from peritoneal dialysis. Electrolytes or medications can be added to the dialysate as needed. For example, antibiotics for peritonitis can be added to the last dwell to allow greater effectiveness with additional contact time with the membrane.

Types of Peritoneal Dialysis

A patient in 2009 has various options in peritoneal dialysis. The main categories are manual versus automated dialysate delivery. CAPD is done by the patient placing fluid in the abdomen and, after the dwell time, draining the fluid. The prescription regulates the contact time which the dialysate fluid has with the membrane and the strength of the dialysate solution which controls ultrafiltration. If done by a machine, CCPD can be performed overnight, allowing the patient greater freedom during the day.

Specific Requirements for Peritoneal Dialysis

What specific clearance should be sought for either CAPD or CCPD is still under debate. Prior guidelines, urging high amounts of clearance with Kt/V of more than 2 have been withdrawn and the 2006 NKF/KDOQI guidelines suggest a minimal Kt/V of 1.7 inclusive of residual renal function based on failure to discern benefit from the greater clearances in the ADMEX and Hong Kong studies. The most recent guidelines (issued in 2006), by the National Kidney Foundation/Kidney Dialysis Outcomes and Quality Initiative, are reflective of the thinking above and suggest inclusion of residual renal function in a desired total KT/V urea of 1.7 weekly in continuous peritoneal dialysis.[17] No trial data is available with automated peritoneal dialysis but the guidelines suggest the same clearances as continuous therapies.

The peritoneal equilibration test (PET) assesses the membrane transport function and categorizes patients into high, low, and average transporters with respect to their glucose and creatinine transportation. Two-thirds of patients were average transporters; the remainder were divided into high and low transport status.[18] Transport characteristics correlate with age in two studies. An association is noted with increasing age and higher transport status at the start of dialysis.[19,20]

Drawbacks

Peritonitis

Peritonitis occurring about once every year is the most frequent cause for catheter loss, loss of membrane and, in the past, discontinuing peritoneal dialysis as a modality for renal replacement therapy.[21,22] Mortality is associated with some organisms more than with others, such as in fungal peritonitis. Techniques and technology have reduced the number of peritonitis infections from 1 in 11 to 1 in 24 or more patient months. The Y system used in combination with the flushing-before-filling concept and the double bag set have decreased the number of peritoneal infections.[23,24] Organisms cultured from active peritonitis cases include gram-positive, gram-negative, fungal, and tuberculous ones. Formation of a biofilm, otherwise known as slime, can cause relapsing peritonitis and is seen more often with *Pseudomonas* and staphylococci.[25] Sclerosing encapsulated peritonitis is a cause of loss of the membrane and moving patients to other modalities of renal replacement.

Protein loss

During peritoneal dialysis there is protein loss into the dialysate and this is of concern, with the background of the CANUSA study showing for each 1 g/dL increase in plasma albumin levels a decrease in risk of mortality by 6%.[26] Attempts to use amino acid solution in addition to other sources of nutrition to minimize protein loss in dialysate have yielded some success.[5] There is no evidence, however, that supports prescription of a specific daily protein intake. Protein intake should be individualized for the patient, taking into account the overall clinical situation, including membrane characteristics. For example, rapid transporters have greater loss of protein into the dialysate compared to other patients.[27] Rapid transporters may need a greater protein intake.

Gastrointestinal complications

Gastrointestinal complications include abdominal hernias, intestinal perforation, and abdominal and thoracic cavity leakage of dialysate solution. Abdominal hernias are a specific problem associated with peritoneal dialysis with the increase in abdominal girth, especially with large volume exchanges. Increased abdominal girth and intra-abdominal pressure, gastric reflux, and slowing of gastric emptying are also reported, along with an increased incidence of chronic back pain. Interestingly, chronic abdominal pain noted on instilling the dialysate solution may be related to the characteristics of the solution: acidic and at an uncomfortable temperature. Suggestions for help include using an addition of bicarbonate to the dialysate, changing the temperature of the dialysate, and slowing the rate of instillation.

Advanced glycosylated end products

AGEs are thought to be toxic and serum levels increase inversely to the glomerular filtration rate. These glucose degradation products are not well removed by either hemodialysis or peritoneal dialysis. For peritoneal dialysis, Zeier *et al.* have postulated that glucose degradation products from peritoneal dialysate solution that are formed during storage may enter the systemic circulation.[28] What toxicity results from absorption from the dialysate is still unclear.

Electrolyte imbalances

An increase in calorie intake with the dialysate with poor glycemic control and weight gain may be a concern in overweight diabetic renal failure patients using higher carbohydrate concentration peritoneal dialysate.

Advantages

Residual renal function

Preservation of residual renal function is better with peritoneal dialysis than with hemodialysis, for unestablished reasons. Among the postulated reasons is that peritoneal dialysis results in a more volume-expanded state and less exposure to nonbiocompatible and proinflammatory tissue. According to several investigators, the rapid changes in volume, electrolytes, and blood pressure that are present during hemodialysis to remove the "incentive" for the remaining nephrons to function are absent with continuous peritoneal dialysis. Interestingly, two studies compared CAPD and CCPD and noted that the continuous therapy provided the greatest preservation in renal residual function, and that the loss of renal function in the intermittent peritoneal dialysis therapies was similar to that in hemodialysis.[29,30] It could be postulated that the more continuous the therapy is, the better residual renal function is preserved.

Cost

The annual expense of treating uremia by peritoneal dialysis in 2004 was about US$20,000 less a year compared with hemodialysis. In a study by Shi *et al.* the unadjusted average medicare expenditure in 2004 dollars for peritoneal dialysis as the first modality of therapy was US$53,277 compared to US$72,189 for hemodialysis, both values with a confidence interval of 95%.[31]

Better blood pressure and anemia control

With peritoneal dialysis, better anemia control with less need for erythropoietin-stimulating agents when compared to hemodialysis is noted. It has also been postulated that there is less stimulation of the immune system with peritoneal dialysis, leading to less inflammation and less anemia.

Other benefits include patient independence seen with a home therapy.

Recent Uses; Innovations in Peritoneal Dialysis Techniques and Technologies

Congestive heart failure

Acute symptom relief and functional improvement along with decrease in hospitalization involving peritoneal dialysis in patients with refractory congestive heart failure and patients without end stage renal disease have been noted in small unrandomized studies.[32]

Solutions

Dialysate containing amino acids to support anabolism has been clinically tested; however, the limiting factor has been acidosis. A combination carbohydrate and amino acid has also been tried in a small number of patients with the intention of promoting protein synthesis.[33] The objective of maximizing ultrafiltration during peritoneal dialysis while decreasing exposure to osmotic agents like glucose and maximizing sodium removal has led to multiple formulations of dialysate. Most recently, the removal of sodium and water with peritoneal dialysis employing a combination of two osmotic dialysate using 2.6% glucose/6.8% icodextrin solutions compared to conventional therapy with either 3.86% glucose or 7.5% icodextrin has been tried by Galach, which revealed increased ultrafiltration due to the additive effects of the solutions.[34]

Convenience

Nonisothermal reactors for the production of pure water from the spent dialysate may in future help with storage of less dialysate.[35] Better storage tanks have been useful as well. In addition, smaller automated machines have helped patients travel, allowing for greater patient autonomy when compared to the past.

The Future of Peritoneal Dialysis

While significant benefits — including preservation of residual renal function, and better control of blood pressure and anemia — are noted, especially in patients unable to tolerate the more aggressive hemodialysis therapies, the benefits weaken quickly over time, with an increase in mortality seen as early as one year after the initiation of renal replacement therapy. The option of peritoneal dialysis has mostly been based on patient lifestyle and socioeconomic rather than clinical factors, even though it is an excellent modality for renal replacement therapy. Underprescribed by suboptimally trained kidney specialists, it remains an underutilized therapy for kidney failure and the number of peritoneal dialysis patients has declined in the past few years. In the near future, we may see an increase in the number of peritoneal dialysis patients for economic reasons as the overall number of kidney disease patients increases while the value of the dollar and the number of dollars spent on health care decrease.

Hopefully, in ten years the dialysis modality whether, it be hemodialysis or peritoneal dialysis, will be a treatment of the past, used only in the acute setting of kidney failure till native kidney recovery occurs or the patient gets a stem cell kidney transplant.

References

1. Teschner M, Heidland A, Klassen A, *et al.* (2004) Goerg ganter: a pioneer of peritoneal dialysis and his tragic academic demise at the hands of the Nazi regime. *J Nephrol* **17**(3): 457–460.
2. Buoncristiani U, Cozzari M, Quintaliani G, *et al.* (1983) Abatement of exogenous peritonitis risk using the Perugia CAPD system. *Dial Transplant* **12**: 14.
3. Majorca R, Cantaluppi A, Ponticelli C, *et al.* (1983) Prospective controlled trial of a Y connector and disinfectant to prevent peritonitis in continuous ambulatory peritoneal dialysis. *Lancet* **2**(8351): 642–644.
4. Balteau P, Peluso F, Zaruba, *et al.* (1991) Design and testing of the Baxter Intergrated Disconnect Systems (IDS). *Perit Dial Int* **11**(2): 131–136.
5. Popovich RP, Moncrief JW, Nolph KD, Ghods AJ, Twardowski ZJ, Pyle WK. (1978) Continuous ambulatory peritoneal dialysis. *Ann Intern Med* **88**(4): 449–456.
6. Boen ST, Mion CM, Curtis FK, Shilipeter G. (1964) Periodic peritoneal dialysis using the repeat puncture technique and an automated cycling machine. *Trans Am Soc Artif Intern Organs* **10**: 409–414.
7. Kopple JD, Bernard D, Messan J, *et al.* (1995) Treatment of malnourished CAPD patients with an amino acid based dialysate. *Kidney Int* **47**: 1148.

8. Paniagua R, Amato D, Vonesh E, Correa Rotter R, Ramos A, Moran J, Mujais S. (2002) *J Am Soc Nephrol* **13**(5): 1307–1320.

9. Lo WK, Ho YW, Li CS, Wong KS, Chan TM, Yu AW, Ng FS, Chen IK. (2003) Effect of Kt/V on survival and clinical outcome in CAPD patients in a randomized prospective study. *Kidney Int* **64**(2): 649–656.

10. USRDS 2008 Annual Data Report.

11. McDonald SP, Marshall MR, Johnson DW, Polkinghorne KR. (2009) Relationship between dialysis modality and mortality. *J Am Soc Neprol* **20**(1): 155–163. Epub December 17, 2008.

12. Jaar BG, Coresh J, Plantinga LC, *et al.* (2005) Comparing the risk for death with peritoneal dialysis and hemodialysis in a national cohort of patients with chronic kidney disease. *Ann Intern Med* **143**(3): 174–183.

13. Mehrotra R, Kermah D, Fried L, Kalantar Zadek K, Khawar O, Norris K, Nissenson A. (2007) Chronic peritoneal dialysis in the US: declining utilization despite improving outcomes. *J Am Soc Nephrol* **18**(10): 2781–2788.

14. Kimmel P, Bosch J. (1991) Effectiveness of renal fellowship training for subsequent clinical practice. *Am J Kidney Dis* **18**(2): 249–256.

15. Carruthers DM, Whishaw JM, Thomas M, Thatcher G. (1996) Planes, kangaroos and the CAPD manual. *Perit Dial Int* **16**(Suppl 1): S452–S454.

16. Carruhters D, Warr K. (2004) Supporting peritoneal dialysis in remote Australia. *Nephrology* **9**(Suppl 4): S129–S133.

17. K/DOQI Clinical Practice Guidelines for peritoneal dialysis adequacy. (2006) *Am J Kidney Dis* **47**(Suppl 4): S1.

18. Twardowski ZJ. (1990) The fast peritoneal equilibration test. *Semin Dial* **3**: 141.

19. Rumpsfeld M, McDonald SP, Purdie DM, *et at.* (2004) Predictors of baseline peritoneal transport status in Australian and New Zealand peritoneal dialysis patients. *Am J Kidney Dis* **43**: 492.

20. Selgas R, Bajo MA, Cirugeda A, *et al.* (2005) Ultrafiltration and the small solute transport at initiation of PD: questioning the paradigm of peritoneal function. *Perit Dial Int* **25**: 68.

21. Schreiber M, Burkart JM, *et al.* (1996) Peritonitis remains the leading cause of transfer from peritoneal dialysis to hemodialysis. *Perit Dial Int.*

22. Woodrow G, Turner JH, Brownjohn AM. (1997) Technique failure in peritoneal dialysis and its impact on patient survival. *Perit Dial Int* **17**(4): 360–364.

23. Daly CD, Campbell MK, MacLeod AM, *et al.* (2001) Do the Y set and double bag systems reduce the incidence of CAPD peritonitis? A systematic review of randomized control trials. *Nephrol Dial Transplant* **16**(2): 341–347.

24. Strippoli GF, Tong A, Johnson D, *et al.* (2004) Catheter related interventions to prevent peritonitis in peritoneal dialysis: A systematic review of randomized control trials. *J Am Soc Nephrol* **15**(10): 2735–2746.

25. Finkelstein ES, Jekel J, Troidle L, *et al.* (2002) Patterns of infection in patients maintained on long term peritoneal dialysis therapy with multiple episodes of peritonitis. *Am J Kidney Dis* **39**(6): 1278–1286.

26. Canada–USA Peritoneal Dialysis Study Group. (1996) Adequacy of dialysis and nutrition in continuous peritoneal dialysis: Association with clinical outcomes. *J Am Soc Nephrol* **7**(2): 198–207.

27. Nolph KD, Moore HL, Prowant B, *et al.* (1993) Continuous ambulatory peritoneal dialysis with a high flux membrane. *ASAIO J* **39**(4): 904–909.

28. Zeier M, Schwenger V, Deppisch R, *et al.* (2003) Glucose degradation products in PD fluids: Do they disappear from the peritoneal cavity and enter the systemic circulation? *Kidney Int* **631**(1): 298–305.

29. Hufnagel G, Michel C, Queffeulou G, *et al.* (1999) The influence of automated peritoneal dialysis on the decrease in residual renal function. *Nephrol Dial Transplant* **14**(5): 1224–1228.

30. Hiroshige K, Yuu K, Soejima M, *et al.* (1996) Rapid decline of residual renal function in patients on automated peritoneal dialysis. *Perit Dial Int* **16**(3): 307–315.

31. Shih YC, Guo A, Just PM, Mujais S. (2005) Impact of initial dialysis modality and modality switches on Medicare expenditures of end stage renal disease patients. *Kidney Int* **68**(1): 319–329.

32. Cnossen N, Kooman JP, Konings CJ, *et al.* (2006) Peritoneal dialysis in patients with congestive heart failure. *Nephrol Dial Transplant* **21**(Suppl 2): ii63–ii66.

33. Tjiong HL, Rietveld T, Wattimena JL, *et al.* (2007) Peritoneal dialysis with solutions containing amino acids plus glucose promotes protein synthesis during oral feeding. *Clin J Am Soc Nephrol* **21**(1): 74–80.

34. Galach M, Werynski A, Waniewski J, Freida P, Lindholm B. (2009) Kinetic analysis of peritoneal fluid and solute transport with combination of glucose and icodextrin as osmotic agents. *Perit Dial Int* **29**(1): 72–80.
35. Diano N, Ettari G, Grano V, *et al.* (2007) Nonisothermal reactors for the production of pure water from peritoneal dialysis waste waters. *Int J Artif Organs* **30**(1): 53–63.

CHAPTER 2

Hemodialysis

Yalemzewd Woredekal*

Introduction

In the last two decades there has been an enormous growth in the number of patients with end stage renal disease (ESRD). The incidence of treated ESRD patients increased rapidly through the 1980s and 1990s: starting from 1980, it increased by 155% by 1990 (217.9 per million) and 295% by 2000 (337.5 per million). During the past few years, the incidence seems to have stabilized and has increased by only 1% since 2001.[1]

Hemodialysis is the most-often-used treatment for ESRD. The United States Renal Data System (USRDS) in 2008 reported that, of the 341,319 prevalence ESRD patients who were receiving renal replacement therapy in 2006, 314,162 (92%) were treated with hemodialysis.[1]

The expenditures for hemodialysis totaled nearly US$17 billion in 2006, while the costs for peritoneal dialysis approached US$1 billion, and those for transplant reached US$1.8 billion, just under 10% of the total sum spent. Expenditure per patient year showed a parallel trend with hemodialysis costs at US$71,889 in 2006, compared to 53,327 and 24,951, respectively, for peritoneal dialysis and transplant.[1]

History of Hemodialysis

The term "dialysis" was first used in 1861, by Thomas Graham, Professor of Chemistry at Anderson's University in Glasgow, Scotland.

* Assistant Professor of Medicine, SUNY–Downstate Medical Center.
Email: ywordekal@aol.com

He noticed that crystalloids were able to diffuse through vegetable parchment coated with albumin that acted as semipermeable membrane. He called this "dialysis." Using this method he was able to extract urea from urine.[2]

In 1913, Abel, Rowntree, and Turner built the first artificial kidney. They passed animal blood from an artery through celloidin tubes that were contained in a glass "jacket." The glass jacket was filled with saline or artificial serum. They called this apparatus an "artificial kidney." Blood was returned into the vein of the animal via another cannula.[2]

In 1943, the first hemodialysis machine used for humans was developed by WJ Kolff and J Berk, from the Netherlands. The rotating drum artificial kidney consisted of 30–40 m of cellophane tubing wrapped around a small drum. The drum was partially immersed in a stationary 100-liter tank holding the dialysate, which was saline solution.

In 1946, Nils Alwall produced the first dialyzer with controlled ultrafiltration. In the early 1950s, the original Kolff rotating drum kidney was modified in Boston to make the Kolff–Brigham kidney and was used to treat renal failure at a few centers and in the Korean War.[2]

For the next decade, hemodialysis was used only to treat acute reversible renal failure because vascular access required repeated surgical insertion of cannulas into the artery and vein, thus limiting the number of treatments that could be carried out.

In 1960, Scribner and coworkers at the University of Washington in Seattle made long-term hemodialysis treatment possible by developing a shunt made up of two plastic tubes (polytetrafluoroethylene (PTFE), one inserted into an artery and one into a vein. After treatment, the circulatory access would be kept open by connecting the two tubes outside the body using a small U-shaped device, which would shunt the blood from the tube in the artery back to the tube in the vein. The Scribner shunt was developed using the newly introduced material, Teflon. With the shunt, it was no longer necessary to make new incisions each time a patient underwent dialysis. In 1962, Scribner started the world's first outpatient dialysis facility.[3]

Six years later, in 1966, Brescia-Cimino developed a forearm fistula, which did not require exteriorized pieces of plastic. This was another major advance for hemodialysis as a long-term treatment for chronic renal failure.[2]

Process of Hemodialysis

Hemodialysis is a process by which solute and fluid are removed from the body. It consists of diffusion and convection. Diffusion refers to the movement of solutes from a compartment in which they are in high concentration to one in which they are in lower concentration along an electrochemical gradient. It is influenced by the blood flow rate, the characteristics of the solute (molecular weight), and the surface area of the membrane. Urea is most commonly chosen as the marker for small molecule diffusion during hemodialysis. Larger molecules are poorly removed by this process.

Convection (ultrafiltration) is a process in which solute is carried along with a fluid across a semipermeable membrane in response to a transmembrane pressure gradient. Ultrafiltration depends upon the pore size of the membrane and the hydrostatic pressure of the blood. It is very effective in removal of fluid.

Hemodialysis Machine

There are five major parts to the hemodialysis machine: dialyzer, blood pump, dialysate pump, safety monitors, and alarm.

(1) *Dialyzer* (artificial kidney). This consists of a blood compartment, a dialysate compartment, and a semipermeable membrane. There are three types of dialyzers:

  (i) *Coil dialyzer*. This was the first to be mass-produced. It had a cellulose coil wrapped around a wire mesh drum. The filtration rate was unpredictable and is no more in use now.

  (ii) *Parallel plate dialyzer*. This uses several plates with ridges and grooves. A semipermeable membrane rests between the grooves. With this dialyzer resistance to blood flow is low and the ultrafiltration rate is controllable and predictable. This kind of dialyzer is rarely used now.

(iii) *Hollow fiber dialyzer*. This type of dialyzer is most commonly used in the USA. It is a cylinder filled with thousands of tiny hollow fibers. Blood flows inside the fibers, and dialysate flows around their outer surface. This dialyzer is compact, easy to handle, and amenable to sterilization and reuse.

(2) *Dialysis membrane*. The three major types of dialysis membrane currently available are:

(i) *Cellulose*. Also called cuprophane, this is a polysaccharide-based membrane obtained from pressed cotton. It has free hydroxyl groups that may enhance reaction with the blood components. These are known to cause complement activation and release of cytokines.

(ii) *Modified cellulose*. This is made by chemical bonding of a material to the free hydroxyl groups at the surface of the cellulose polymer. These consist mainly of various degrees of substitution of the hydroxyl groups on the cellulose backbone. The most common type is cellulose acetate, in which acetate replaces most of the hydroxyl group.

(iii) *Synthetic membrane*. This is made by the addition of synthetic material such as diethylaminethyl to liquefied cellulose during the formation. This type of dialysis membrane is most commonly used in the USA. There are varieties of synthetic membrane, such as polyacrylonitrile, polysulfone, and acrylnitrile-sodium methallysulfonate (AN-69). These membranes are believed to be more biocompatible and cause less complement activation and cytokine release. Membrane composition has been associated with dialyzer performance. High-efficiency dialyzers can be made from all types of membrane material, and high-flux dialyzers are manufactured from modified cellulose and synthetic membrane with equal performance.

(3) *Dialysis machine.* The blood pump moves the blood from the patient through the arterial line into the dialyzer and back to the patient through the venous line. The speed of the blood pump can be adjusted from 200 to 600 ml/min. The dialysate pump uses suction to move the dialysate into the dialyzer and removes the ultrafiltrate from the dialyzer. The flow rate of the dialysate can be adjusted, and is usually set between 500 and 800 ml/min. The arterial and venous pressures are monitored during the dialysis treatment. The arterial pressure is measured before the blood pump to detect excessive suction of blood, and the venous pressure is measured after the dialyzer to detect high resistance on the venous side of the access. The safety guards of the dialysis machine include the air detector, the blood leak detector, and the measurement of the conductivity and temperature of the dialysate. If any one of these safety guards malfunctions, the alarm system will be triggered so that action can be taken by the dialysis personnel.

Water Treatment System for Hemodialysis

Water purification for preparation of dialysate fluid is a major part of hemodialysis treatment. Hemodialysis patients are vulnerable to a large amount of contaminants in water used for hemodialysis treatment. The average water intake by healthy individuals is 10–14 liters per week, while hemodialysis patients are exposed to 340–400 liters per week — more than 25 times the exposure.

The quality of the water contributes very significantly to morbidity and life-threatening reactions in dialysis patients in both acute and long-term consequences.[4]

A water purification process consists of different steps: use of sediment filters for removal of coarse particles, water softener for removal of calcium and magnesium by exchanging them for sodium ions, and carbon adsorption to remove chloramines from the water as this contaminant can cause hemolysis if it gets into the bloodstream. The final processing system consists of reverse osmosis and deionization.

Reverse osmosis (RO) uses high pressure to force water across semipermeable membrane. It is very effective in removing bacteria, viruses, endotoxins, and ionic and nonionic contaminants.

Deionization uses ion exchange resins to remove ionic contaminants from water by exchanging hydrogen ions from cation and hydroxyl from anions. It is usually employed as a secondary or backup purification step following RO. If RO is malfunctioning or is insufficient to provide water for the requisite quality, deionization can be used.[5]

When is the Time to Initiate Hemodialysis Treatment?

Traditionally, nephrologists have used various approaches in deciding on the proper timing of initiation of dialysis. Clinical signs and symptoms along with observation of laboratory data are an important part of the decision-making process. In 1997, the National Kidney Foundation–Dialysis Outcomes Quality Initiative (NKF–DOQI) publication outlined guidelines for initiation of dialysis.[6] Two separate laboratory criteria were considered to be used as a threshold below which initiation of dialysis should be contemplated. The first is the residual renal function, as measured in units of Kt/V urea. The guideline states that initiation of dialysis should be considered when the residual renal function gets Kt/V below 2 L/week. This threshold is extrapolated from morbidity and mortality study of peritoneal dialysis patients.[7] The CANUSA (Canada–USA) study, a prospective, multicenter cohort study of 680 incident peritoneal dialysis patients, showed an inverse relationship between small solute clearance and mortality rate. Over a two-year period, every 0.1 U/week increase in the total Kt/V was found to correspond to a 6% decrease in the relative risk of death. The total Kt/V and creatinine clearance values which corresponded to a 78% two-year survival rate were 2.1 L/week and 70 L/1.73 m2/week, respectively.

The second laboratory value for initiation of dialysis is the normalized protein equivalent of nitrogen appearance (nPNA). This value is a measure of protein excretion, and, indirectly, a measurement of protein intake. It is well known that uremic patients have a lower daily protein intake, which causes them to be in a negative nitrogen balance. Initiation of dialysis is recommended for patients with a value of nPNA less than 0.8 g/kg/day. In addition to the above laboratory values, clinical signs and symptoms of individual patients should be considered to make the appropriate decision.

There are specific indications for starting dialysis early for patients with chronic renal insufficiency. They include intractable fluid overload that is not responding to diuretics, intractable hyperkalemia, and metabolic acidosis unresponsive to medical therapy.

Dialysis Vascular Access

The discussion about different options of renal placement therapy should be started once the estimated glomerular filtration rate (eGFR) is less than 30 ml/min. If the patient chooses hemodialysis, the veins in the nondominant arm should not be used for venipuncture. Placement of the central line in the subclavian vein should also be avoided.

There are three types of vascular access that can be used for hemodialysis treatment.

(1) *Arteriovenous fistula.* This is the preferred type of vascular access. A fistula is created by connecting an artery directly to a vein, often in the forearm (radial–cephalic fistula) or the upper arm (brachial–cephalic vein fistula or brachia–basilica vein fistula). The AV fistula requires advance planning, because a fistula takes time to mature after it is created. It has a weaker tendency to form clots and be infected than the other type of vascular access. For patients who do not have visible veins, venous mapping will help the surgeon to choose an appropriate vein for creating the fistula.

(2) *Arteriovenous graft.* This is created only if it is not possible to create a fistula because the patient's veins are too small to be used. It is made by using a synthetic tube to connect an artery to a vein. The tube can be used repeatedly for needle placement and blood access during hemodialysis. A graft does not need to be developed as a fistula, so it can be used sooner after

placement, usually after two or three weeks. Compared to the AV fistula, the graft has more problems with clotting and infection.

(3) *Central venous catheter.* This is placed as a temporary access for those patients whose renal function deteriorates fast before a permanent access is placed or before it matures. The catheter is placed in the internal jugular vein on the opposite side of the permanent access that has been placed in. It can be used immediately after its position is confirmed by radiology. The catheter has two chambers to allow a two-way flow of blood. Central venous catheters are most likely to develop infections and clotting problems.

Monitoring of Vascular Access

Vascular access dysfunction in hemodialysis patients is common and results in inadequate dialysis and an increased risk of thrombosis. There is evidence that several methods of access monitoring can predict the presence of hemodynamically significant stenosis which leads to access thrombosis. The approaches to access assessment include physical examination of the access, access recirculation during dialysis, measurements of flow and pressure for structural abnormality, and measurement of dialysis adequacy. Physical examination is a simple and quick method for assessment of vascular access. The presence of abnormal findings or a change in the findings should prompt a more detailed evaluation of the vascular access. For example, persistent pulsation throughout the graft with little or no detectable thrill is highly predictive of an outflow stenosis. Nursing and technical staff should be encouraged to examine the access before needle placement at each dialysis session. Doppler ultrasound and ultrasound dilution can be used to measure access blood flow. Color-flow Doppler studies are also able to detect stenosis of vascular access and venous outflow. The ideal frequency for monitoring vascular access is not known, but it has to be individualized. Patients with a previous history of angioplasty of their access may need to have frequent surveillance of their accesses.

Hemodialysis Treatment

Hemodialysis treatment can be delivered in-center or at home. It can be given in a conventional way, or as short daily or long nocturnal hemodialysis.

(1) *In-center hemodialysis.* This is the most common type of treatment in the USA. Patients come to a dialysis center and receive their treatment three times a week, 3–4 h per session. In this setup the treatment is given by a nurse or a patient care technician with nursing supervision. Some centers are also self-care centers, where patients participate in their care. The patients are trained to set up their machines and at times to cannulate their vascular access as well. The dialysis staff monitor the treatment.

(2) *Home hemodialysis.* In the early 1970s, home hemodialysis was the preferred treatment, but currently it accounts for less than 1% of all hemodialysis treatment in the USA.[1] Home hemodialysis treatment can be done as conventional hemodialysis (three times a week, 3–5 h per session), or short daily (six days a week, 2–3 h per session) or long nocturnal dialysis (six nights a week, 6–8 h per session). It has been shown that home hemodialysis provides better patient survival, better control of hypertension with fewer antihypertensive medications, and better quality of life and rehabilitation.[8,9]

Dialysis Prescription

A dialysis prescription includes the type of dialyzer, frequency and duration of dialysis treatment, blood flow, dialysate flow, composition of dialysate (K, Ca, bicarbonate), use of anticoagulation, and estimated dry weight. The prescription is aimed at delivering an acceptable urea clearance. The urea clearance can be adjusted by using a different dialyzer clearance or changing the duration of dialysis. The usual clinical practice is to be careful in the prescription of the initial dialysis by limiting dialysis time, blood flow, volume removed, and urea clearance to avoid disequilibrium syndrome.

Complications Related to Hemodialysis

(1) *Intradialytic hypotension.* This is a frequent complication seen in hemodialysis patients. The factors involved in intradialytic hypotension include hypovolemia (when the refilling rate is slower than the ultrafiltration rate), diastolic dysfunction (limiting cardiac output with a decrease in ventricular filling pressure due to hypovolemia), autonomic dysfunction (limiting vasoconstriction), and dialysis composition such as low calcium concentration. Meal ingestion may also be involved in the genesis of hypotension, by decreasing blood volume and reducing vasoconstriction of the resistance vessels in the splanchnic area, with the consequence of an increased venous capacitance in this area and reduced venous return.[10] Many of the hypotensive episodes can be prevented by prescribing an accurate dry weight. The dry weight is usually established clinically, with inaccurate targets set. Different methods have been used to estimate the dry weight accurately: (i) ultrasonic measurement of the IVC diameter after dialysis, because equilibration of IVC due to plasma volume change occurs only after a period of time; this is not a practical method; (ii) measurement of ANP (atria natriuretic peptide) correlates with dry weight in study populations, but not in individuals; (iii) evaluation of transthoracic or segmental bioelectric impedance measurements. Sympatomimetic agents, such as midodrine and the norepinephrine precursor L-dopa, have been successfully used to prevent intradialytic hypotension.[11,12]

(2) *Muscle cramps.* These are likely to be related to changes in muscle perfusion that occur in response to ultrafiltration during hemodialysis. In addition to fluid shift, electrolyte and acid-base changes may also contribute to these symptoms. Immediate treatment for muscle cramps includes interruption or slowing of the ultrafiltration rate and administration of hypertonic saline. Preventive measures are also aimed at stabilizing the hemodynamic status by carefully reassessing the dry weight, and counseling the patient to try not to reduce interdialytic weight gain.

(3) *Febrile reactions.* Endotoxins are the major players in causing pyrogenic reaction. Fever, chills, headache, myalgia, and hemodynamic instability are the characteristics of pyrogenic reaction. Endotoxins are liposaccharides with a high molecular weight, derived from the outer membrane of gram-negative bacteria. The main source of contamination is the dialysate because of contaminated water and a bicarbonate bath. The major consequence of endotoxins is the release of pyrogenic cytokines from monocytes and endothelial cells mediating a cascade of clinical events.

References

1. United States Renal Data System. (2008) USRDS 2008 annual data report: atlas of kidney disease and end-stage renal disease in the United States. National Institutes of Health, National Institute of Diabetes and Digestive and Kidney diseases, Bethesda, MD.
2. Maher JF. (1989) Replacement of renal function by dialysis, in *Textbook of Dialysis.*
3. Blagg CR, Ing TS, Berry D, Kjellstrand CM. (2004) The history and rationale of daily and nighly hemodialysis. *Contrib Nephrol* **145**: 1–9.
4. Arnow PM, Bland LA, Garcia-Houchins S, Fridkin S, Fellner SK. (1994) An outbreak of fatal fluoride intoxication in long-term hemodialysis unit. *Ann Int Med* **121**: 337.
5. Cappelli G, Ravera F, Ricardi M, *et al.* (2005) Water treatment for hemodialysis: a 2005 update. *Contrib Nephrol* **149**: 42–50.
6. NKF–DOQI Clinical Practice Guidelines for Peritoneal Dialysis Adequacy. (1997) National Kidney Foundation, New York.
7. Canada–USA (CANUSA) Peritoneal Dialysis Study Group. (1996) Adequacy of dialysis and nutrition in continuous peritoneal dialysis: association with clinical outcomes. *J Am Soc Nephrol* **7**: 198–207.
8. McGregor D, Buttimore A, Robson R, *et al.* (2000) Thirty years of universal home hemodialysis in Christchurch. *NZ Med J* **113**: 27.
9. Chan CT, Floras JS, Miller JA, Richardson RM, Pierratos AL. (2002) Regression of left ventricular hypertrophy after conversion to nocturnal hemodialysis. *Kidney Int* **61**: 2235–2239.

10. Levin NW, Ronco C. (2002) Complications during hemodialysis, in *Textbook of Dialysis Therapy*, 3rd ed.
11. Prakash S, Garg AX, Heidentheim AP, House AA. (2004) Midodrine appears to be safe and effective for dialysis-induced hypotension: a systematic review. *Nephrol Dial Transplant* **19**(10): 2553–2558.
12. Hoecen H, Abu-Alfa AK, Mahnensmith R, Perazella MA. (2002) Hemodynamics in patients with intradialytic hypotension treated with cool dialysate or midodrine. *Am J Kidney Dis* **39**(1): 102–107.

CHAPTER 3

Kidney Transplantation

*Fasika Tedla**

Introduction

In 1901, Sir William Osler in his famous textbook of medicine wrote of chronic kidney disease (or "Bright's disease," as it was then called):

> Chronic Bright's disease is an incurable affection, and the anatomical conditions on which it depends are quite as much beyond the reach of medicine as wrinkled skin or gray hair.[1]

a hopeless prognosis which was the fate of many until Willem Kolff invented the artificial kidney in 1944, converting a uniformly fatal disease to a treatable one.[2] Although kidney transplantation was technically feasible in animals and humans earlier than the introduction of dialysis, the immunologic barriers to transplantation and the means of overcoming them were not understood until much later.[3–5]

By the end of 2006, over 350,000 kidney failure patients were receiving either hemodialysis or peritoneal dialysis and approximately 150,000 lived with functioning renal allografts in the United States.[6] Kidney transplantation, once a mode of treatment fraught with complications and high mortality, has now become the preferred treatment for kidney failure. After briefly reviewing the early developments that made transplantation possible, this chapter

*Medical Director of Kidney Transplantation, SUNY Health Science Center at Brooklyn, New York, USA. Email: fasika.tedla@downstate.edu

discusses: recent trends in outcome; evaluation of donors and recipients; important aspects of transplant immunology; and immunosuppression and posttransplant care.

Historical Perspective

Mankind's age-old fascination with the ability to replace organs, narrated often in religious or mythical contexts, started to take a scientific form when the seemingly parallel worlds of tumor biology, genetics, immunology and surgery intersected toward the end of the first half of the 20th century.[3] A broad timeline of the milestones is shown in Table 1.

The murine genetic locus that determines tumor transplantability (H-2) was discovered by Snell and Gorer in 1948.[7] In the 1960s and 1970s, H-2 was found to be the analog of the human leukocyte antigen (HLA) system and its role in antigen presentation was defined (discovered by Dausset, Zinkernagel and Doherty).[4]

Tumor researchers and surgeons alike had described intense lymphocytic infiltrates in rejected tissue. Murphy even demonstrated that lymphocyte depletion by X-irradiation inhibits tumor rejection.[3]

Table 1. Milestones in Transplantation*

Milestone	Year
Technique of vascular anastomosis	1902
Successful human corneal allograft	1906
Inhibition of rejection of tumor transplants by X-irradiation	1910s
Immune and genetic basis of resistance to tumor transplants	1910s
First deceased donor renal transplant in humans	1936
Immune basis of transplant rejection	1944
Discovery of mouse histocompatibility gene (H-2)	1948
Clonal deletion theory	1949
Evidence for clonal deletion theory and tolerance	1950s
First successful kidney transplant	1954
First description of human leukocyte antigen	1958
Use of azathioprine in transplantation	1962

*Summarized from Refs. 3–5.

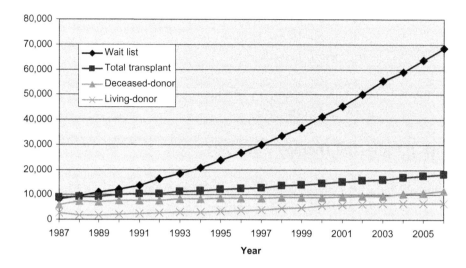

Fig. 1. Number of patients on the waiting list and who received living or deceased donor kidney transplant from 1987 to 2006. (*Data from United States Renal Data System*, 2008.[6])

2006 as compared to 1987, but the number of patients on the waiting list increased by more than eightfold in the same period. Contributing to this divergence is the limited availability of kidneys for transplantation, the increasing prevalence of end-stage renal disease (ESRD) and the relaxation of criteria for transplant candidacy.

The mortality of wait-listed patients has increased, with a larger proportion of older patients having more comorbidities. According to the latest USRDS data, adults younger than 44, who in 1990 constituted nearly two-thirds of wait-listed patients, represented only 30.1% of this population in 2006. In the same period, the unadjusted mortality for wait-listed dialysis patients rose from 46.4 to 71.7 per 1000 patient-years and the median waiting time nearly tripled.[6] These trends have stimulated innovative approaches to expanding the donor pool, and better utilizing the currently available kidneys, as discussed below.

Patient Survival

Improvement in transplant medicine has yielded the current one-year patient survival of 95% compared to 60% in 1970, despite older and sicker patients being transplanted.[13–15] Now cardiovascular disease is the leading cause of death — a shift from the early days of renal transplantation, when most patients succumbed to infections.[15–17] In a landmark study by Wolfe *et al.*, recipients of deceased kidney transplants were found to have better long-term survival than patients who remained on the waiting list and this advantage was observed for all age groups and categories of renal diseases, although younger patients and those with diabetes gained the most survival benefit.[18]

Graft Survival

The introduction of cyclosporine into clinical practice in the 1980s increased one-year graft survival from 50–60% to over 70%.[19,20] Current three-drug immunosuppression regimens consisting of a calcineurin inhibitor (CNI) (cyclosporine or tacrolimus), antimetabolite (azathioprine or mycophenolate) and corticosteroids attain one-year graft survival in excess of 90%.[6,21] While improvements in short-term survival and reduction in rates of acute rejection have occurred, only modest change is observed in long-term graft outcome when graft survival depends on a complex interplay between immunologic factors, drug toxicity and nonimmunologic risk factors for kidney disease, such as hypertension and diabetes.

Living donor renal transplants confer better graft survival and function than deceased donor transplants, even with genetically unrelated donors.[6,22,23] In addition to donor source, other factors that adversely affect graft survival are prior sensitization,[24] acute rejection,[25] delayed graft function[26] and longer duration of dialysis prior to transplantation.[27,28] Patients who undergo pre-emptive renal transplantation appear to have better graft and patient survival in uncontrolled studies.[28–30] Short of randomized controlled trials, it is difficult to distinguish whether this is a direct effect or related to unique characteristics of the subset of renal failure patients who receive pre-emptive renal transplant.

Approaches to Increasing the Donor Pool

The creative measures implemented to deal with the critical shortage of kidneys for transplantation include increasing use of kidneys from extended criteria donors, donation after cardiac death, increasing deceased donor consent and donation, desensitization to transplant across immunologic barriers, and donor exchange programs.

Extended criteria donor (ECD) kidneys are from donors older than 60 or aged 50–59, with two of the following characteristics: terminal creatinine of 1.5 mg/dL or higher; death due to cerebrovascular accidents; a history of hypertension.

Donation after cardiac death (DCD) is said to occur when organs are procured after life support is withdrawn to allow cessation of cardiac activity; DCD kidneys therefore suffer longer warm ischemia than those procured under standard criteria donation (SCD). Kidney transplants with DCD kidneys have been increasing rapidly in the last decade and now represent 10% of all deceased donor kidney transplants in the US. Similarly, use of ECD kidneys has been increasing since nationwide adoption of ECD guidelines in 2002, accounting for approximately 20% of all deceased donor kidney transplants in 2006.[6] Although ECD kidneys are associated with higher rates of graft loss than SCD kidneys, they still result in better patient survival than remaining on the waiting list.[31] This is especially true of elderly patients, who may have a shorter life expectancy than the average waiting time for SCD kidneys.[31,32]

The Health Resources and Services Administration, a branch of the United States Department of Health and Human Services, introduced the Organ Donation Breakthrough Collaboration in 2003 and, together with transplant centers, organ procurement organizations and donor hospitals, addressed barriers to consenting to donation and utilization of recovered organs, leading to an increase in rates of consent for deceased donation and organ recovery.[33] Blood group incompatibility and presence of donor-specific anti-HLA antibodies present major barriers to transplantation. Desensitization, the attenuation of antibody response against the donor to a degree that allows transplantation, has been achieved with administration of high-dose intravenous immune globulin (IVIG) or a combination of low-dose IVIG and plasmapheresis. In patients with high antibody titers, adjunctive therapy with splenectomy or, more recently, the monoclonal anti-CD20 antibody rituximab — a selective anti-B-lymphocyte agent — may be necessary. Patients who otherwise would have been unable to undergo transplantation have been successfully transplanted using these protocols, albeit with acute rejection rates as high as 50%.[34,35] Similar encouraging results are attained in donor exchange programs, in which a pool of incompatible donor-recipient pairs are matched in such a way that exchange of the donors would allow transplantation between compatible individuals.[36,37]

Global Trends

Worldwide, more than 400,000 of the nearly 1.8 million patients with ESRD who were receiving some form of renal replacement therapy (RRT) in 2004 had functioning renal allografts.[38] These numbers underestimate the true global prevalence of ESRD, since treatment rates of uremia vary widely even among industrialized nations, and appear to be dictated by the economic strength and reimbursement policies of a particular country.[39] The global incidence and prevalence of chronic kidney disease (CKD) are rising along with the increase in diabetes and ageing of the world population. Illustrating this awareness are recent publications by national and international professional organizations that highlight the importance of CKD as a global public health threat and outline guidelines for its prevention and treatment.[40,41]

Evaluation for Kidney Donation

Transmission of infection or malignancy is a major concern in all forms of transplantation. Besides evaluation for human immunodeficiency virus (HIV), hepatitis B and C viruses, cytomegalovirus (CMV), human T-cell lymphotropic virus (HTLV) and untreated bacterial infections, the panel of infectious agents tested for should be tailored to the local epidemiology of infectious diseases in both donor and recipient. For instance, testing for Chagas disease is recommended in South America, as are tests for parasitic infections such as amoebiasis and strongyloidiasis in countries where these diseases are endemic. The global nature of disease transmission is highlighted by recent reports of rabies and Chagas disease transmitted by solid organ transplants.[42,43]

Active overt malignancy is a contraindication for organ donation. Earlier reports of tumor transmission with transplanted organs[44,45] resulted in patients with a history of cancer traditionally being excluded from donation, even though experience with transplants performed using organs from individuals with a history of cancer has shown that the risk of tumor transmission is very low, and that mortality from donor-related tumors is even lower. In an analysis of registry data, the deceased-donor-related tumor rate was 0.04%, and mortality due to deceased donor tumors was 0.007%.[46] It is notable that the majority (71.5%) of organ donors with histories of tumors other than nonmelanoma skin or primary CNS cancer had tumor-free intervals greater than five years.[47] In general, the likelihood of tumor transmission diminishes as the disease-free interval increases. Current guidelines for living donor evaluation recommend only age-appropriate cancer screening for those without a history of cancer.

Evaluation of potential living kidney donors covers several areas other than disease transmission, as shown in Table 2. Surgery for organ donation is unique in that the procedure is performed for the benefit of another individual. As a result, the evaluation and consent processes of living kidney donation require additional safeguards to ensure that the potential donor has a full grasp of the risks of donation and, within the constraints of patient confidentiality, the expected outcome of kidney transplantation for the recipient. Most transplant centers have separate medical teams to evaluate donors and recipients, so as to avoid conflicts of interest.

Table 2.   Aspects of Living Donor Evaluation that are Different from Deceased Kidney Donation

Psychosocial:	Motivation
	Evidence of psychopathology
Consent for:	Evaluation
	Surgery
Surgical Evaluation:	Vascular anatomy
	Urologic anatomy
Medical Evaluation:	Standard preoperative evaluation
	Renal function
	Risk factors for kidney disease

As unrelated donors become a significant proportion of all living donors, thorough assessment of the motivation of the donor and the power relationship between donor and recipient has assumed increasing importance.[48] The ideal donor should have no psychiatric disorder or substance abuse and be able to freely donate the organ. Extensive education about the transplant process, and separate consents for evaluation and surgery, are needed for all donors. In addition to standard preoperative assessment, donors need to know if they have any renal disease, risk factors for renal disease or anatomical aberrations that impact on suitability for kidney donation. The short-term risks of kidney donation are low. In a national survey, mortality from uninephrectomy was estimated at 0.03%, whereas reoperation was required in 0.4–1% of cases.[49] Laparoscopic nephrectomy is associated with less morbidity than open nephrectomy, without an increase in complication rates.

Several studies examining the long-term risks of kidney donation have shown that the procedure appears to be safe for donors, although there may be a mild increase in blood pressure or proteinuria. Risk of kidney disease and mortality were not found to be increased as compared to that of the general population or, in some studies, matched controls.[50–55] While these observations are encouraging, they should be interpreted with caution, for several reasons: most studies had a small sample size; were largely single-center; had retrospective design; and spanned long periods of time, during which patient selection criteria evolved.

Evaluation of Kidney Transplant Candidates

The process of evaluation assesses medical suitability and also educates the patient about posttransplant care. As with evaluation of potential living donors, a multidisciplinary team weighs the risks and benefits of transplantation for each patient. The American Society of Transplantation has guidelines to aid in the evaluation of patients who do not have any of the absolute contraindications shown in Table 3.[56] Selected aspects of the pretransplant workup are discussed below.

Cardiovascular disease

Cardiovascular disease is common and is a leading cause of death among dialysis patients and renal transplant recipients.[15,57] Which is the best diagnostic strategy and whether coronary revascularization improves survival remain controversial.[58] Current guidelines recommend noninvasive testing for patients with coronary risk factors, and

Table 3.   Absolute Contraindications for Kidney Transplantation

Active infection
Active malignancy
Untreated psychiatric disorder
Active substance abuse
Refractory nonadherence
Limited potential for rehabilitation
Irreversible major organ failure*
Primary oxalosis*

*If not eligible for multiorgan transplant.

coronary angiography for patients who have symptomatic angina or abnormal results on noninvasive testing.[56,58] Management of cerebrovascular and peripheral vascular disease is similar to that for the general population.

Infections

All treatable infections should be eradicated prior to kidney transplantation and since the number of possible infections to be considered is large the decision to test for specific diseases should be guided by the local epidemiology of infections in a given population. As transplant recipients have reduced response to immunization, it is preferable to administer all necessary vaccines before transplantation.

Patients with ESRD may have a higher risk of developing tuberculosis than the general population.[59] Tuberculin skin testing and chest x-rays are done routinely on transplant candidates. Whether treatment of latent tuberculosis reduces the risk of reactivation tuberculosis after transplant is controversial. However, most transplant centers treat patients having latent tuberculosis with isoniazid before and/or after transplant, especially those with risk factors for reactivation, such as residence in endemic areas, exposure to patients with active tuberculosis, or evidence of previous tuberculosis by either history or radiography.

Serologic tests for HIV, hepatitis C virus (HCV), hepatitis B virus (HBV), syphilis, HTLV and CMV are standard components of the pre-transplant evaluation. Once considered a contraindication, HIV infection does not preclude candidacy for kidney transplantation if certain criteria are met. These criteria include adherence to antiretroviral therapy, stable CD4+ T-lymphocyte count ≥ 200, undetectable viral load and absence of a history of opportunistic infections.[60,61]

Chronic hepatitis secondary to HCV and/or HBV poses a significant challenge in the evaluation of renal transplant candidates.[62,63] As transaminase levels do not correlate with the degree of hepatic injury or viral replication, quantitation of viral copies and liver biopsy are often required. Patients with histologic evidence of cirrhosis or bridging necrosis tend to decompensate after transplantation and should get combined liver–kidney transplants when eligible. There are limited data on how to manage those with milder degrees of liver damage. Interferon therapy appears to have a higher risk of side effects in ESRD patients and of rejection after transplantation.

Malignancy

Immunosuppression predisposes to certain kinds of cancers and may adversely affect the course of pre-existing cancers. For renal transplant candidates who do not have a history of malignancy, only age-appropriate cancer screening is recommended. Based on experience from tumor registries of transplant recipients, disease-free waiting periods of different lengths have been recommended for specific malignancies for patients with a history of cancer.[56] In general, waiting periods of 2–5 years are considered appropriate for most solid tumors; patients with *in situ* carcinomas do not require a waiting period as long as they are properly treated. The decision to proceed with kidney transplantation in a specific patient should be done in consultation with an oncologist.

Disease Recurrence

Some renal disorders tend to recur in allografts and the likelihood of recurrence varies with the specific disease process.[56] Primary oxalosis and type II membranoproliferative glomerulonephritis (MPGN) almost always recur after transplantation. Graft loss in MPGN, however, is much less than that in oxalosis, which occurs in nearly all recipients. Focal segmental glomerulosclerosis, IgA nephropathy, hemolytic–uremic syndrome/thrombotic thrombocytopenic purpura and renal vasculitides have intermediate risks of recurrence. Approximately 3–5% of patients with Alport syndrome may develop antiglomerular basement membrane antibody–mediated glomerulonephritis in their allografts. Since recurrence does not portend graft loss in the majority of cases, the diagnosis of most of these disorders does not imply ineligibility for renal transplantation. However, the risk of recurrence should be discussed during pretransplant evaluation, especially in cases involving living donors.

Histocompatibility

The presence of ABO incompatibility or preformed cytotoxic anti-HLA antibodies is considered a major barrier to successful transplantation. Well-matched kidney transplants have longer graft survival than their poorly matched counterparts, but excellent outcomes can be attained even in those with less perfect HLA matching using modern immunosuppression. More sensitive molecular and solid-phase techniques now augment older serologic methods of HLA typing and detection of anti-HLA antibodies. These developments allow identification of HLA antigens, and the specificities and levels of anti-HLA antibodies — details that help sensitized patients avoid exposure to recall antigens.[64]

Immunosuppression

Basics of alloreactivity

The ability of the immune system to differentiate self from nonself occurs during early development, when potentially self-reactive clones of T-lymphocytes are eliminated. Unlike antibodies, which bind both protein and nonprotein antigens, T-lymphocytes respond only to peptides bound to one of two types of major histocompatibility complex (MHC) molecules. Class I MHC molecules, expressed on the surface of all nucleated cells, present endogenous peptides, whereas class II MHC molecules are restricted to antigen-presenting cells — specialized cells that process foreign protein antigens.

Similar to immunoglobulins, the T-cell receptor (TCR) is a heterodimer of two polypeptides that have highly variable regions for antigen binding. Activation of T-lymphocytes requires two simultaneous signals: the TCR engages an MHC molecule carrying a foreign peptide or altered endogenous peptide; and the T-cell and APC interact through additional surface molecules. Presentation of antigen to T-lymphocytes in the absence of the latter, called costimulation, results in anergy instead of activation, and eventual death by apoptosis. More recently, it has become clear that there are coinhibitory as well as costimulatory signals, and the final outcome appears to depend on which pathway predominates in a given state.[65,66] The dissection of these pathways is a very active area of research at present.

Concurrent presence of TCR engagement and positive costimulation recruits several other molecules that trigger intracellular signaling and T-cell activation. These molecules, such as CD3 and ζ-associated protein, are closely associated with the TCR. Their cytoplasmic domains have tyrosine kinase activity and in turn activate several intracellular pathways involved in regulation of many transcription factors and cytokines. Figure 2 schematically depicts one of the best-characterized components of this cascade — the calcineurin pathway. Phosphorylation of ZAP-70 (ζ-associated protein 70 kDa) leads to activation of phospholipase Cγ1 (PLC γ1), which catalyzes the hydrolysis of phosphatidylinositol diphosphate into diacylglycerol (DAG) and inositol triphosphate. Calcium–calmodulin complex, formed when the calcium-dependent protein calmodulin binds with DAG-released calcium, then activates the cytoplasmic phosphatase calcineurin. The target of the potent immunosuppressants cyclosporine and tacrolimus, calcineurin then activates the nuclear factor of activated T-cells (NFAT), a key regulator of the transcription of interleukin 2 (IL-2) and other cytokines. These cytokines control complex processes involved in activation and proliferation of immune cells.

Immunosuppressive Agents

Calcineurin inhibitors

The cornerstone of modern immunosuppression, this class of drugs consists of cyclosporine and tacrolimus, and interferes with the calcineurin pathway described above. In randomized trials, long-term

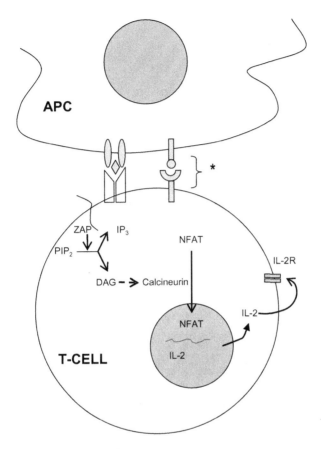

Fig. 2. Signaling in T-lymphocyte activation. APC = antigen-presenting cell; DAG = diacylglycerol; IL-2 = interleukin 2; IL-2R = IL-2 receptor; IP_3 = inositol triphosphate; NFAT = nuclear factor of activated T-cells; PIP_2 = phosphatidylinositol bisphosphate; ZAP = ζ-associated protein; * = costimulatory/inhibitory molecules.

graft survival did not differ between the two agents, but tacrolimus was associated with less acute rejection.[21,67,68] These drugs share several side effects: both agents are nephrotoxic; hypertension, hyperlipidemia and gout are more common with cyclosporine, while diabetes and neurotoxicity are more frequent with tacrolimus. Cyclosporine causes gingival hyperplasia, hirsutism and nail dystrophy. Tacrolimus, may cause hair loss.

Antimetabolites

Antimetabolites interfere with the synthesis of nucleic acids. Two antimetabolites, mycophenolic acid and azathioprine, are currently used in transplantation. Mycophenolic acid is a competitive inhibitor of inosine monophosphate dehydrogenase (IMPDH), a rate-limiting enzyme in the *de novo* synthesis of purines. Since lymphocytes are more dependent on this pathway than other tissues, which have an alternative salvage pathway to generate purine nucleotides, mycophenolic acid is a relatively selective inhibitor of lymphocytes. It is marketed in two formulations, one of which is enteric-coated. In randomized trials, there was no significant difference in the frequency of gastrointestinal side effects between the two formulations.[69,70] In both formulations the common adverse effects include gastrointestinal disturbance, leucopenia and thrombocytopenia. Azathioprine is a purine analog that interferes with transcription, with the main side effect of bone marrow suppression and, rarely, cholestatic hepatitis or pancreatitis. Its use has declined since the introduction of the more effective mycophenolate mofetil.[71] In patients taking allopurinol, azathioprine should be discontinued or its dosage reduced to 25–50% to avoid profound bone marrow suppression.

Corticosteroids

Corticosteroids have well-known anti-inflammatory, antifibrotic, and several metabolic effects. Due to side effects, minimization or avoidance of steroids has drawn interest and, although some short-term studies have shown satisfactory outcomes, results have not been uniform or confirmed in long-term trials.[72]

mTOR inhibitors

There are two agents that exert their immunosuppressive effect by inhibiting a kinase — mammalian target of rapamycin (mTOR) — involved in cell cycle regulation. Sirolimus (Rapamune®, also called rapamycin) is available in the United States; Everolimus, which differs from the former in that it has a shorter half-life, is not. Impaired wound healing, hyperlipidemia and bone marrow suppression are major side effects. As the two agents do not have direct nephrotoxicity, they have been used in calcineurin inhibitor minimization protocols or as a substitute for CNIs. Short-term studies suggest that mTOR inhibitors may help preserve graft function, but long-term data are limited.[73,74]

Monoclonal and polyclonal antibodies

Since the 1970s, antibody preparations have been used as immunosuppressants. Polyclonal antibodies are generated by immunizing horses or rabbits with human lymphoid tissue and are composed of cytotoxic antibodies against lymphocytes and other cell types. Thymoglobulin (rabbit antibody against thymocytes) is the agent widely used in the United States.

OKT3, a murine monoclonal antibody directed against the CD3 T-cell marker, was the first monoclonal to be used in clinical medicine. Since its introduction in 1987, two humanized monoclonal antibodies against the IL-2 receptor, basiliximab and daclizumab, have been developed. Alemtuzumab, a humanized anti-CD52 antibody approved for treatment of chronic lymphocytic leukemia, has also been employed in transplantation.

Thymoglobulin, OKT3 and alemtuzumab deplete circulating lymphocytes, whereas basiliximab and daclizumab are nondepleting agents. Unlike the humanized monoclonal antibodies, xenogeneic antibodies (thymoglobulin and OKT3) may induce immune response in the recipient, and repeated treatment may result in lack of efficacy.

Immunosuppression protocols

Conventional immunosuppression currently consists of a CNI, an antimetabolite or mTOR inhibitor and low-dose corticosteroids. Some centers also administer induction — the intensification of immunosuppression immediately after transplantation using one of the antibodies described above — especially in high-risk patients or those considered for steroid avoidance/withdrawal.

Posttransplant Care

As renal transplant recipients become older and live longer, management of coexisting comorbidities has assumed increasing importance.[75,76] In addition, immunosuppression is associated with new medical conditions or exacerbation of pre-existing ones. The incidence of new-onset diabetes is estimated at 13.4%, although it appears to be much higher in those patients who have additional risk factors. These factors include race (African-Americans and Hispanics), older age, treatment with tacrolimus, pretransplant glucose intolerance, infection with hepatitis C and obesity.

Renal transplant recipients have fracture rates that exceed 4–5 times that in age-matched individuals in the general population.[75,77] Persistent hyperparathyroidism, vitamin D deficiency, corticosteroids, hypophosphatemia, hypomagnesemia and age-related osteoporosis all play a role in the pathogenesis of bone disease after transplantation.

Treatment of acute rejection

Acute rejection is the single most important preventable factor that portends inferior long-term outcome[25] and the highest risk is in the first year after transplantation, especially the first 3–6 months. Late rejections should raise the possibility of nonadherence or drug interactions that reduce exposure to immunosuppressive medications. The most common manifestation of acute rejection is usually a rise in serum creatinine. Once alternative diagnoses such as volume depletion or obstruction are excluded, allograft biopsy should be performed to confirm the diagnosis. Treatment with high-dose corticosteroids usually reverses most episodes of cell-mediated rejection, but when it fails or biopsy shows high-grade rejection, use of OKT3 or thymoglobulin is appropriate.

Infections

The overall risk of infection after transplantation is a function of the degree of immunosuppression, the virulence of the organism and the level of exposure. Since transplant recipients cannot mount a robust inflammatory response, it is important to maintain a high index of suspicion for a wide spectrum of infectious agents. Unusual opportunistic infections should alert clinicians to the possibility of overimmunosuppression even when drug levels are within the expected range.

Cytomegalovirus (CMV) infection is one of the most important complications of renal transplantation. The availability of effective prophylaxis has reduced morbidity and mortality from CMV disease among kidney transplant recipients.[78] Risk of posttransplant CMV disease is related to recipient and donor serostatus at the time of transplantation, and the degree of immunosuppression posttransplant.[79] Seronegative transplant recipients who receive kidneys from seropositive donors have a much higher risk of primary CMV disease than seropositive recipients who get organs from either seronegative or seropositive donors; transplants in which both the donor and the recipient are seronegative have the lowest risk, so much so that some centers choose not to give prophylaxis to this group. Prophylaxis is usually given for the first 100 days after transplantation, or during periods of intensification of immunosuppression.

Malignancy

Renal transplant recipients appear to have a higher risk than the general population for most cancers.[80,81] Compared to patients on the kidney waiting list, transplant recipients develop more oral, skin, renal and lymphoid malignancies, and Kaposi's sarcoma.

Posttransplant lymphoproliferative disorder (PTLD) represents a spectrum of neoplastic processes, ranging from benign polyclonal hyperplasia to aggressive high-grade lymphoma. It is the most common tumor after nonmelanoma skin cancer among transplant patients. Predominantly of B-cell origin, its overall incidence is estimated at 1–5% among solid organ transplant recipients, but is much higher in Epstein–Barr virus (EBV)–negative pediatric recipients of organs from EBV-positive donors.[82] Although some studies have found association with specific immunosuppressive agents, the risk of PTLD is most likely related to the overall degree of immunosuppression. Once diagnosed, patients require reduction of immunosuppression. Patients with high-grade lymphoma are usually treated with chemotherapy regimens that include rituximab.

Future Directions

Advances in molecular biology are uncovering new potential targets for immunosuppression. Small-molecule or biological agents that block intracellular signaling pathways, costimulation, adhesion molecules and the complement cascade are at various stages of development.[83] The search for noninvasive markers of rejection will likely accelerate as new tools of investigation enrich those that are currently available.[84,85]

While these lines of investigation will undoubtedly advance the science and practice of renal transplantation, they do not directly address the critical shortage of organs. If tissue engineering techniques overcome the immunological barrier between species, xenotransplantation may make the current debate about regulated markets for living donor kidneys only of historical interest.[86–88]

Summary

Kidney transplantation has evolved from a fledgling discipline practiced by a select few to a mainstream treatment modality in as little as 50 years. In the process, both society and medical professionals have had to grapple with clinical, legal and ethical issues that did not exist before. The history of the development of transplantation biology and medicine illustrates the value of collaboration between clinicians and scientists in diverse fields of study. If this history is any guide, the surest prediction one can make is that the current march of molecular biology and genomic medicine will probably take us to places we cannot yet imagine.

References

1. Osler W. (1901) *The Principles and Practice of Medicine*, 4th ed. D Appleton, New York.
2. Kolff W, Berk H, Welle M, van der Ley A, van Djik E, van Noordwijk J. (1944) The artificial kidney: a dialyser with a great area. *Acta Med Scand* **177**: 121–134.
3. Silverstein A. (1989) *A History of Immunology*. Academic, San Diego.
4. Brent L. (1997) A History of Transplantation Immunology. Academic, San Diego.
5. Stefoni S, Campieri C, Donati G, Orlandi V. (2004) The history of clinical renal transplant. *J Nephrol* **17**(3): 475–478.
6. US Renal Data System, USRDS. (2008) Annual Data Report: Atlas of Chronic Kidney Disease and End-Stage Renal Disease in the United States (National Institutes of Health, Bethesda, MD).
7. Gorer P, Lyman S, Snell G. (1948) Studies on the genetic and antigenic basis of tumor transplantation: Linkage between a histocompatibility gene and "Fused" in mice. *Proc R Soc London B* **135**: 499–505.
8. Medawar PB. (1944) The behaviour and fate of skin autografts and skin homografts in rabbits: A report to the War Wounds Committee of the Medical Research Council. *J Anat* **78**(Pt 5): 176–199.
9. Merrill JP, Murray JE, Harrison JH, Guild WR. (1956) Successful homo-transplantation of the human kidney between identical twins. *J Am Med Assoc* **160**(4): 277–282.
10. Schwartz R, Stack J, Dameshek W. (1958) Effect of 6-mercaptopurine on antibody production. *Proc Soc Exp Biol Med* **99**(1): 164–167.
11. Calne RY. (1960) The rejection of renal homografts: Inhibition in dogs by 6-mercaptopurine. *Lancet* **1**(7121): 417–418.
12. Calne RY, Alexandre GP, Murray JE. (1962) A study of the effects of drugs in prolonging survival of homologous renal transplants in dogs. *Ann N Y Acad Sci* **99**: 743–761.

13. Morris PJ. (2004) Transplantation — a medical miracle of the 20th century. *N Engl J Med* **351**(26): 2678–2680.

14. Vincenti F. (2004) A decade of progress in kidney transplantation. *Transplantation* **77**(9 Suppl): S52–S61.

15. Briggs JD. (2001) Causes of death after renal transplantation. *Nephrol Dial Transplant* **16**(8): 1545–1549.

16. Adams PL. (2006) Long-term patient survival: Strategies to improve overall health. *Am J Kidney Dis* **47**(4 Suppl 2): S65–S85.

17. Howard RJ, Patton PR, Reed AI, *et al.* (2002) The changing causes of graft loss and death after kidney transplantation. *Transplantation* **73**(12): 1923–1928.

18. Wolfe RA, Ashby VB, Milford EL, *et al.* (1999) Comparison of mortality in all patients on dialysis, patients on dialysis awaiting transplantation, and recipients of a first cadaveric transplant. *N Engl J Med* **341**(23): 1725–1730.

19. The Canadian Multicentre Transplant Study Group. (1986) A randomized clinical trial of cyclosporine in cadaveric renal transplantation: Analysis at three years. *N Engl J Med* **314**(19): 1219–1225.

20. Ponticelli C, Minetti L, Di Palo FQ, *et al.* (1988) The Milan clinical trial with cyclosporine in cadaveric renal transplantation: A three-year follow-up. *Transplantation* **45**(5): 908–913.

21. Pirsch JD, Miller J, Deierhoi MH, Vincenti F, Filo RS. FK506 Kidney Transplant Study Group. (1997) A comparison of tacrolimus (FK506) and cyclosporine for immunosuppression after cadaveric renal transplantation. *Transplantation* **63**(7): 977–983.

22. Terasaki PI, Cecka JM, Gjertson DW, Takemoto S. (1995) High survival rates of kidney transplants from spousal and living unrelated donors. *N Engl J Med* **333**(6): 333–336.

23. Gjertson DW, Cecka JM. (2000) Living unrelated donor kidney transplantation. *Kidney Int* **58**(2): 491–499.

24. Opelz G. (2005) Non-HLA transplantation immunity revealed by lymphocytotoxic antibodies. *Lancet* **365**(9470): 1570–1576.

25. Hariharan S, Johnson CP, Bresnahan BA, Taranto SE, McIntosh MJ, Stablein D. (2000) Improved graft survival after renal transplantation in the United States, 1988 to 1996. *N Engl J Med* **342**(9): 605–612.

26. Shoskes DA, Cecka JM. (1998) Deleterious effects of delayed graft function in cadaveric renal transplant recipients independent of acute rejection. *Transplantation* **66**(12): 1697–1701.
27. Meier-Kriesche HU, Port FK, Ojo AO, *et al.* (2000) Effect of waiting time on renal transplant outcome. *Kidney Int* **58**(3): 1311–1317.
28. Meier-Kriesche HU, Kaplan B. (2002) Waiting time on dialysis as the strongest modifiable risk factor for renal transplant outcomes: A paired donor kidney analysis. *Transplantation* **74**(10): 1377–1381.
29. Kasiske BL, Snyder JJ, Matas AJ, Ellison MD, Gill JS, Kausz AT. (2002) Preemptive kidney transplantation: The advantage and the advantaged. *J Am Soc Nephrol* **13**(5): 1358–1364.
30. Mange KC, Joffe MM, Feldman HI. (2001) Effect of the use or nonuse of long-term dialysis on the subsequent survival of renal transplants from living donors. *N Engl J Med* **344**(10): 726–731.
31. Ojo AO, Hanson JA, Meier-Kriesche H, *et al.* (2001) Survival in recipients of marginal cadaveric donor kidneys compared with other recipients and wait-listed transplant candidates. *J Am Soc Nephrol* **12**(3): 589–597.
32. Sung RS, Guidinger MK, Leichtman AB, *et al.* (2007) Impact of the expanded criteria donor allocation system on candidates for and recipients of expanded criteria donor kidneys. *Transplantation* **84**(9): 1138–1144.
33. Sung RS, Galloway J, Tuttle-Newhall JE, *et al.* (2008) Organ donation and utilization in the United States, 1997–2006. *Am J Transplant* **8**(4 Pt 2): 922–934.
34. Jordan SC, Peng A, Vo AA. (2009) Therapeutic strategies in management of the highly HLA-sensitized and ABO-incompatible transplant recipients. *Contrib Nephrol* **162**: 13–26.
35. Vo AA, Lukovsky M, Toyoda M, *et al.* (2008) Rituximab and intravenous immune globulin for desensitization during renal transplantation. *N Engl J Med* **359**(3): 242–251.
36. Hanto RL, Reitsma W, Delmonico FL. (2008) The development of a successful multiregional kidney paired donation program. *Transplantation* **86**(12): 1744–1748.
37. de Klerk M, Witvliet MD, Haase-Kromwijk BJ, Claas FH, Weimar W. (2008) Hurdles, barriers, and successes of a national living donor kidney exchange program. *Transplantation* **86**(12): 1749–1753.

38. Grassmann A, Gioberge S, Moeller S, Brown G. (2005) ESRD patients in 2004: Global overview of patient numbers, treatment modalities and associated trends. *Nephrol Dial Transplant* **20**(12): 2587–2593.

39. Friedman EA. (2003) Restating the obvious: The world can't afford American health care. *ASAIO J* **49**(5): 507–509.

40. Levey AS, Atkins R, Coresh J, *et al.* (2007) Chronic kidney disease as a global public health problem: Approaches and initiatives — a position statement from Kidney Disease Improving Global Outcomes. *Kidney Int* **72**(3): 247–259.

41. Davis CL, Harmon WE, Himmelfarb J, *et al.* (2008) World Kidney Day 2008: Think globally, speak locally. *J Am Soc Nephrol* **19**(3): 413–416.

42. Chagas disease after organ transplantation — United States. (2001) *MMWR Morb Mortal Wkly Rep* **51**(10): 210–212.

43. Srinivasan A, Burton EC, Kuehnert MJ, *et al.* (2005) Transmission of rabies virus from an organ donor to four transplant recipients. *N Engl J Med* **352**(11): 1103–1111.

44. Wilson RE, Penn I. (1975) Fate of tumors transplanted with a renal allograft. *Transplant Proc* **7**(2): 327–331.

45. Penn I. (1997) Transmission of cancer from organ donors. *Ann Transplant* **2**(4): 7–12.

46. Myron Kauffman H, McBride MA, Cherikh WS, Spain PC, Marks WH, Roza AM. (2002) Transplant tumor registry: Donor-related malignancies. *Transplantation* **74**(3): 358–362.

47. Kauffman HM, McBride MA, Delmonico FL. (2000) First report of the United Network for Organ Sharing Transplant Tumor Registry: Donors with a history of cancer. *Transplantation* **70**(12): 1747–1751.

48. Dew MA, Jacobs CL, Jowsey SG, Hanto R, Miller C, Delmonico FL. (2007) Guidelines for the psychosocial evaluation of living unrelated kidney donors in the United States. *Am J Transplant* **7**(5): 1047–1054.

49. Matas AJ, Bartlett ST, Leichtman AB, Delmonico FL. (2003) Morbidity and mortality after living kidney donation, 1999–2001: Survey of United States transplant centers. *Am J Transplant* **3**(7): 830–834.

50. Hakim RM, Goldszer RC, Brenner BM. (1984) Hypertension and proteinuria: Long-term sequelae of uninephrectomy in humans. *Kidney Int* **25**(6): 930–936.

51. Talseth T, Fauchald P, Skrede S, *et al.* (1986) Long-term blood pressure and renal function in kidney donors. *Kidney Int* **29**(5): 1072–1076.
52. Najarian JS, Chavers BM, McHugh LE, Matas AJ. (1992) 20 years or more of follow-up of living kidney donors. *Lancet* **340**(8823): 807–810.
53. Ibrahim HN, Foley R, Tan L, *et al.* (2009) Long-term consequences of kidney donation. *N Engl J Med* **360**(5): 459–469.
54. Narkun-Burgess DM, Nolan CR, Norman JE, Page WF, Miller PL, Meyer TW. (1993) Forty-five year follow-up after uninephrectomy. *Kidney Int* **43**(5): 1110–1115.
55. Kasiske BL, Ma JZ, Louis TA, Swan SK. (1995) Long-term effects of reduced renal mass in humans. *Kidney Int* **48**(3): 814–819.
56. Kasiske BL, Cangro CB, Hariharan S, *et al.* (2001) The evaluation of renal transplantation candidates: Clinical practice guidelines. *Am J Transplant* **1**(Suppl 2): 3–95.
57. Foley RN, Parfrey PS, Sarnak MJ. (1998) Clinical epidemiology of cardiovascular disease in chronic renal disease. *Am J Kidney Dis* **32**(5 Suppl 3): S112–S119.
58. Pilmore H. (2006) Cardiac assessment for renal transplantation. *Am J Transplant* **6**(4): 659–665.
59. Chia S, Karim M, Elwood RK, FitzGerald JM. (1998) Risk of tuberculosis in dialysis patients: A population-based study. *Int J Tuberc Lung Dis* **2**(12): 989–991.
60. Kumar MS, Sierka DR, Damask AM, *et al.* (2005) Safety and success of kidney transplantation and concomitant immunosuppression in HIV-positive patients. *Kidney Int* **67**(4): 1622–1629.
61. Qiu J, Terasaki PI, Waki K, Cai J, Gjertson DW. (2006) HIV-positive renal recipients can achieve survival rates similar to those of HIV-negative patients. *Transplantation* **81**(12): 1658–1661.
62. Fabrizi F, Martin P, Ponticelli C. (2002) Hepatitis B virus and renal transplantation. *Nephron* **90**(3): 241–251.
63. Terrault NA, Adey DB. (2007) The kidney transplant recipient with hepatitis C infection: Pre- and posttransplantation treatment. *Clin J Am Soc Nephrol* **2**(3): 563–575.
64. Tait BD, Hudson F, Cantwell L, *et al.* (2009) Review article: Luminex technology for HLA antibody detection in organ transplantation. *Nephrology (Carlton)* **14**(2): 247–254.

65. Kroczek RA, Mages HW, Hutloff A. (2004) Emerging paradigms of T-cell co-stimulation. *Curr Opin Immunol* **16**(3): 321–327.

66. Trikudanathan S, Sayegh MH. (2007) The evolution of the immunobiology of co-stimulatory pathways: Clinical implications. *Clin Exp Rheumatol* **25**(5 Suppl 46): S12–S21.

67. Margreiter R. (2002) Efficacy and safety of tacrolimus compared with cyclosporine microemulsion in renal transplantation: A randomised multicentre study. *Lancet* **359**(9308): 741–746.

68. Johnson C, Ahsan N, Gonwa T, *et al.* (2000) Randomized trial of tacrolimus (Prograf) in combination with azathioprine or mycophenolate mofetil versus cyclosporine (Neoral) with mycophenolate mofetil after cadaveric kidney transplantation. *Transplantation* **69**(5): 834–841.

69. Budde K, Curtis J, Knoll G, *et al.* (2004) Enteric-coated mycophenolate sodium can be safely administered in maintenance renal transplant patients: Results of a 1-year study. *Am J Transplant* **4**(2): 237–243.

70. Salvadori M, Holzer H, de Mattos A, *et al.* (2004) Enteric-coated mycophenolate sodium is therapeutically equivalent to mycophenolate mofetil in *de novo* renal transplant patients. *Am J Transplant* **4**(2): 231–236.

71. Sollinger HW, US Renal Transplant Mycophenolate Mofetil Study Group. (1995) Mycophenolate mofetil for the prevention of acute rejection in primary cadaveric renal allograft recipients. *Transplantation* **60**(3): 225–232.

72. Augustine JJ, Hricik DE. (2006) Steroid sparing in kidney transplantation: Changing paradigms, improving outcomes, and remaining questions. *Clin J Am Soc Nephrol* **1**(5): 1080–1089.

73. Kreis H, Oberbauer R, Campistol JM, *et al.* (2004) Long-term benefits with sirolimus-based therapy after early cyclosporine withdrawal. *J Am Soc Nephrol* **15**(3): 809–817.

74. Webster AC, Lee VW, Chapman JR, Craig JC. (2006) Target of rapamycin inhibitors (sirolimus and everolimus) for primary immunosuppression of kidney transplant recipients: A systematic review and meta-analysis of randomized trials. *Transplantation* **81**(9): 1234–1248.

75. Salifu MO, Tedla F, Markell MS. (2005) Management of the well renal transplant recipient: Outpatient surveillance and treatment recommendations. *Semin Dial* **18**(6): 520–528.

76. Tedla F, Hayashi R, McFarlane SI, Salifu MO. (2007) Hypertension after renal transplant. *J Clin Hypertens (Greenwich)* **9**(7): 538–545.

77. Kunzendorf U, Kramer BK, Arns W, *et al.* (2008) Bone disease after renal transplantation. *Nephrol Dial Transplant* **23**(2): 450–458.

78. Paya C, Humar A, Dominguez E, *et al.* (2004) Efficacy and safety of valganciclovir vs. oral ganciclovir for prevention of cytomegalovirus disease in solid organ transplant recipients. *Am J Transplant* **4**(4): 611–620.

79. Davis CL. (1990) The prevention of cytomegalovirus disease in renal transplantation. *Am J Kidney Dis* **16**(3): 175–188.

80. Kasiske BL, Snyder JJ, Gilbertson DT, Wang C. (2004) Cancer after kidney transplantation in the United States. *Am J Transplant* **4**(6): 905–913.

81. Zafar SY, Howell DN, Gockerman JP. (2008) Malignancy after solid organ transplantation: An overview. *Oncologist* **13**(7): 769–778.

82. Paya CV, Fung JJ, Nalesnik MA, *et al.* (1999) ASTS/ASTP EBV-PTLD Task Force and The Mayo Clinic Organized International Consensus Development Meeting. (1999) Epstein-Barr virus-induced posttransplant lymphoproliferative disorders. *Transplantation* **68**(10): 1517–1525.

83. Vincenti F, Kirk AD. (2008) What's next in the pipeline. *Am J Transplant* **8**(10): 1972–1981.

84. Anglicheau D, Suthanthiran M. (2008) Noninvasive prediction of organ graft rejection and outcome using gene expression patterns. *Transplantation* **86**(2): 192–199.

85. Quintana LF, Sole-Gonzalez A, Kalko SG, *et al.* (2009) Urine proteomics to detect biomarkers for chronic allograft dysfunction. *J Am Soc Nephrol* **20**(2): 428–435.

86. Ogle B, Cascalho M, Platt JL. (2004) Fusion of approaches to the treatment of organ failure. *Am J Transplant* **4**(Suppl 6): 74–77.

87. Friedman EA, Friedman AL. (2006) Payment for donor kidneys: Pros and cons. *Kidney Int* **69**(6): 960–962.

88. Danovitch GM, Delmonico FL. (2008) The prohibition of kidney sales and organ markets should remain. *Curr Opin Organ Transplant* **13**(4): 386–394.

CHAPTER 4

Home Hemodialysis: Present and Future Therapies

*Barbara G. Delano**

Introduction

The present and future of home hemodialysis cannot be discussed without examining the past. Home hemodialysis is defined as dialysis performed in the patient's home. Ideally the patient performs the treatment by himself or herself with or without a helper or assistant. In some circumstances a paid nurse or technician may perform the dialysis. In this chapter we will explore the reasons for the early growth of home hemodialysis, consider reasons for the decline, and discuss our feelings about the possible re-emergence of home hemodialysis as a vibrant, important tool in the treatment of end stage renal disease (ESRD). We will also discuss the benefits and problems with the therapy and finally comment on the exciting new field of more frequent home hemodialysis.

Early History

Many scientific advances occur because of work that has previously been done by others. So too in medicine; occasionally a new therapy will develop in several places at approximately the same time. This is what happened in home hemodialysis. After reports of successful

_____

*Professor of Medicine, Professor of Public Health, Director of Home Dialysis Program, State University of New York–Downstate Medical Center, USA.

chronic dialysis, first in the hospital and then in "satellite" units,[1,2] the next logical question was whether or not this could be performed in the patient's home. To be able to do that would extend the limited resources to others and reduce the cost. Thus, almost simultaneously, hemodialysis in the home was reported by Merrill and coworkers in Boston,[3] Curtis *et al.* in Seattle,[4] and Baillod and Shaldon in England.[5] The impetus for this was largely financial.[6,7] With limited insurance coverage (if any) for this treatment, the move into the home was less costly by virtue of the fact that the labor costs were assumed by the patients and their families. In addition, there was limited space in the few dialysis units that existed and admission was frequently determined by a committee deciding "who shall live and who shall die."[8] While financial factors were the original stimulus for home treatment, it soon became evident that for some patients the independence, flexibility and freedom of receiving treatment at home became of paramount importance. In addition, with time, it became clear that home hemodialysis offered a survival as well as other benefits (see below). Because of these factors home hemodialysis expanded, eventually accounting for 40% of all hemodialysis treatments in the USA in 1972.[9]

Perhaps an illustration of the role home hemodialysis played in the past can be examined from the history of our unit at Downstate Medical Center–Kings County Hospital. The unit began as an offspring of one of the first federally funded demonstration units for chronic dialysis. The location was in an inner-city hospital serving a largely indigent population. The first patient was trained in 1969. By 1976, 78 patients had successfully completed training and 50 were dialyzing at home. The seven-year cumulative mortality was 13%.[10] As the early dialysis machines required a responsible adult to be the patient's partner, the ability to place someone at home was somewhat limited, particularly in our urban area, because of lack of a dialysis helper. To address this concern and increase the number of patients dialyzing at home, in 1978 HCFA Department of Health and Human Services started a demonstration project supplying paid helpers for dialysis patients. Under this project we increased the number of patients, so that in 1986, 84 patients were actively receiving hemodialysis at home. The paid aide program was not without its problems. The use of a paid helper meant that a schedule had to be followed and the flexibility of tailoring the dialysis treatments to suit one's lifestyle was lost. In addition, there were occasional conflicts between the helper and the patient or the patient's family.[11]

From this high of 84 active home patients, a decline in the number of our patients being treated at home began. This was not unique to us, as home hemodialysis nationally declined starting with the passage of HR-1, Public Law 92-603 in 1973. That law extended almost universal Medicare coverage to patients receiving hemodialysis regardless of age.[12] While this was a landmark occurrence for patients with chronic kidney disease in our country, it had a negative effect on home hemodialysis, and by 1996 less that 1% of United States residents were on home hemodialysis (Fig. 1). The major reason was that by virtually eliminating any concerns about cost, the inclusion criteria for dialysis patients greatly expanded to include those not previously accepted, particularly patients with systemic diseases and the aged. Forty-eight percent of incident

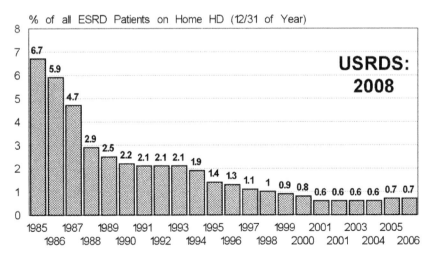

Fig. 1. Percent prevalent home hemodialysis patients.

dialysis patients in 2006 were 65 years of age or older and 45% had diabetes listed as the etiology of their renal disease.[13] These older, sicker patients were less suitable for treatment at home in part because of their many comorbid conditions. In addition, with payment for dialysis patients assured by the federal government, there was a proliferation of free-standing satellite units, many of which were for-profit. There was thus a financial incentive for the outpatient units to have all their chairs filled, and in some units patients were not encouraged to go home.

The next nail in the coffin of home dialysis was the introduction of chronic ambulatory peritoneal dialysis by Moncrief and Popovich in the late 1970s.[14] The ease of training patients for peritoneal dialysis and the ability of the patients to perform the therapy without a helper, as well as the lack of any durable medical equipment, soon led to peritoneal dialysis being the usual home therapy for those independent patients. An additional factor in the decline of home hemodialysis was that the number of programs offering training in home hemodialysis and the number of patients on the therapy decreased. Of the more that 100 nephrology training programs, fewer than 10% offer training in home treatment, and thus trainees have little opportunity to learn about this therapy and then do not feel comfortable offering it to patients.[15]

Benefits of Home Hemodialysis

Survival

In addition to having the ability to tailor the dialysis treatment time to one's convenience, there quickly were reported several medical benefits accruing to patients dialyzing at home. Perhaps the most important benefit reported was that of improved patient survival. Delano reported a 58% ten-year survival of patients on home dialysis[16] and Woods, using United States Renal Data System (USRDS) data, reported that the relative risk of death for home hemodialysis patients was 0.63, corrected as much as possible for variables like age, diabetes and other comorbid conditions.[7] Of course, short of a randomly controlled trial (ethically impossible to perform), in which patients are assigned to one therapy or the other, the true difference in survival cannot be known; however, an interesting case-control study by Saner *et al.* helps to answer the question. For each home hemodialysis patient trained in their unit, the authors, using a retrospective chart review, selected an in-center patient matched for gender, age, therapy duration and etiology of renal disease. There was no difference found in the Kahn comorbidity index, hypertension, smoking, history of myocardial infarction, etc. The 5-, 10- and 20-year survival rates were 93%, 72% and 34% for patients on home hemodialysis and 64%, 48% and 23% for those receiving center dialysis.[17]

Other advantages

Other advantages of early home hemodialysis included the fact that patients were less likely to contact hepatitis and more likely to participate in full-time activities or to be gainfully employed.[18] Home patients state that they like the sense of "control" and the ability to adjust their dialysis schedule to their needs. They also save time traveling to and from the dialysis unit.[19]

Cost

Cost data are very hard to evaluate, as actual cost and reimbursement are frequently interchanged. Using Medicare reimbursement for satellite dialysis and the cost of training for home hemodialysis obtained from our hospital business office, we estimated that for our center, after a period of 14.4 months, the excess costs of training for home were followed by a saving of US$7472.40 per patient per year.[6] In a more recent paper analyzing cost and health-related quality of life for home hemodialysis and satellite self-care patients, no significant difference in cost was found; however, the distribution of the costs varied. Home hemodialysis patients had higher direct costs of the procedure, in part because they had on average longer and more frequent sessions. This additional cost was balanced by lower travel costs. There was no difference in the health-related quality of life.[20]

Table 1. Mean Annual Per Patient Costs of Dialytic Therapy in Finland

Modality	Cost (Finnish dollars)
In-center dialysis	78,000
CCPD	51,000
Self-care	48,000
CAPD	42,000
HHD	37,000

CCPD = automated peritoneal dialysis; CAPD = chronic ambulatory peritoneal dialysis; HHD = home hemodialysis.

From Ref. 45.

Table 1 compares mean annual cost per patient for various dialysis treatments in Finland.

In a theoretical cost analysis using a multiple-cohort Markov model, Howard and coworkers estimated that increasing home hemodialysis to the highest rates achieved at some Australian centers could save 46.6 million Australian dollars by 2010.[21]

Barriers to Home Hemodialysis

There are many barriers to home hemodialysis that must be overcome for successful training and therapy. There is a lack of awareness among patients about home hemodialysis, in part because of the discomfort with the therapy among nephrologists who have not had much opportunity to see patients on this therapy, as stated above. In addition, according to Mehrotra *et al.* 36% of patients did not have previous contact with a nephrologist until dialysis was imminent, and only 12% were offered this as an option.[22] Patient-related factors include much comorbidity, belief that they can be better cared for in a hospital, fear of needles and self-cannulation, and, particularly in inner-city areas, lack of a suitable partner.[23]

Present and Future Home Hemodialysis

Home hemodialysis at present accounts for less than 1% of all patients receiving hemodialysis in this country and it has an uneven distribution. Illinois and Florida have the highest incidence of home patients at 29% and 26%, respectively.[13] However, the recent interest in more frequent hemodialysis, short daily dialysis and nocturnal hemodialysis being therapies most conveniently performed at home has led to great interest and the possible beginning of resurgence in home hemodialysis.

Indeed, the NIH has sponsored an International Quotidian Dialysis Registry to prospectively study those patients performing more frequent dialysis. As of July 2008, there were approximately 2000 patients from Canada, the United States and Australia registered.[24]

The modern age of more frequent hemodialysis was restarted by Udall and coworkers as slow nocturnal home hemodialysis in 1994. The patients were dialyzed with a low blood flow using an external jugular catheter. At that time the patients had eight hours of treatment during sleep, six days per week.[25] In 1997, Dr. Lockridge at Lynchburg, Virginia started a nocturnal home hemodialysis program, and he had trained more that 75 patients at the end of 2007, with very encouraging results. In an attempt to see what penetration more frequent dialysis had made in the United States, this group sent a questionnaire to the largest dialysis providers as well as midlevel units to determine the number of patients using this therapy, in December 2007. Of a total of 3764 patients, 841 were doing conventional home hemodialysis, 2396 were on short daily, and 527 were performing nocturnal treatment either every other night or more that five times per week.[26]

Reported Benefits of More Frequent Dialysis

One of the almost-universal findings about patients undergoing nocturnal hemodialysis is improvement in blood pressure and or less antihypertensive medications required for control.[27–29]

The most consistent finding in studies of nocturnal home hemo-dialysis is improvement in serum phosphorous, occasionally to levels at which supplementation has to be given. Kooienga measured the total weekly phosphorus removed with nocturnal home dialysis and found that the amount was more than twice that of conventional thrice-weekly dialysis (4985 mg/wk +/– 1827 vs. 2347 mg/wk +/– 697), resulting in a significantly lower serum phosphorus level in patients despite an increase in dietary protein and phosphorous intake.[30] Nessim *et al.* found a similar decrease in serum phosphorus levels and also noticed an increase in 25 and 1,25 vitamin D levels without a change in PTH. They postulated that the normalization of serum PO_4 may improve 1-alpha-hydroxylation, thus enhancing substrate-dependent generation of vitamin D in those patients.[31]

Another consistent finding in studies of nocturnal hemodialysis is an increase in serum hemoglobin levels or a decrease in erythro-poietin doses, or both.[32] In an elegant study, Chan *et al.* obtained data suggesting that nocturnal hemodialysis improves anemia by facilitating the growth of hematopoietic cells. Plasma samples from 16 stable patients who underwent a period of frequent nocturnal treatment were more likely to support the frequency and size of erythroid (BFU-E) and granulocytic (CFU-GM) colony growth in culture compared to the plasma from the same patients obtained during conventional hemodialysis.[33] Other benefits reported include improvement in sleep apnea[34] and improvement in lipid profiles.[35]

Of interest is a recent study in which no overall improvement in quality of life was found in a group of 52 patients undergoing nocturnal hemodialysis compared to conventional treatment. This study, however, was just six months in duration and it is possible that a longer study will have other results.[36]

Several of the above medical benefits have also been found for short daily dialysis. In addition, short daily dialysis has been reported to have a marked effect on cardiovascular risk factors. In one study, despite similar baseline measurements of the left ventricular mass index (LVMI) by echocardiogram, C-reactive protein (CRP), calcium, phosphorous and the erythropoietin resistance index (ERI), after one year patients assigned to short daily dialysis had a 30% reduction in the LVMI, while the conventionally dialyzed patients had no change. In addition, the short daily dialysis patients' CRP decreased from a baseline of 1.22 to 0.05 mg/dl, while conventionally treated patients had a slight increase in the level.[37]

Phosphorus control with short daily dialysis has not been as successful as with long overnight treatment. In a crossover study that used patients as their own control, Williams *et al.* found an improvement in blood pressure control and less use of erythropoietin, but no change in bone mineral control.[38] On the other hand, Takayuki did find significantly lower serum phosphorous levels in a group of 26 patients receiving short daily dialysis compared to 51 controls after a 12-month period ($p = 0.01$).[39]

While there is a lot of enthusiasm about daily dialysis, it is clear that all the answers are not yet in. Suri *et al.* did a systematic review of articles written. Twenty-five of 233 articles met their inclusion criteria. This represented 268 patients with an age range of 41–64 years. Fifty percent of those patients were doing daily dialysis at home and more that 90% had fistulas. As the different reports varied widely, so did the results. The most consistent finding was a decrease in blood pressure that was found in 10 of the 11 studies that examined it. There was no significant decrease in phosphorus in 6 of the 8 studies and the hemoglobin increased in 7 of 11. The median survival rate for patients treated at home (for 3–24 months) was 93% (range 85–100%).[40] Chazot and Guillaume found better survival for dialysis patients treated at home compared to daily in-center patients, and both had a superior 10-year survival over conventionally treated patients. They do, however, caution that there may be a downside to increasing dialysis frequency: no randomized clinical trial has yet demonstrated a clinical advantage; the economic advantages are not clear; patients may be concerned about their safety at home or difficulty in sleeping while on nocturnal home hemodialysis, and there is the question of patients' willingness and compliance.[41] In one study of 126 patients, 44% said that they would not choose daily dialysis regardless of the benefits and 56% said that they would if medical benefits could be demonstrated.[42] On the other hand,

Pierratos has recently opined that despite the many reported benefits of more frequent hemodialysis, as yet there does not seem to be
a major move in that direction.[43]

In addition to the usual barrier to home dialysis, the more intensive therapies raise questions about the cost of more frequent
treatments and reimbursement issues. There is also concern about
increased use of vascular access, although studies have not shown
any detrimental effects to date.[44] Again, according to Dr. Pierratos,
a major change will occur when the medical benefits are clear, the
technique is simple enough for widespread use, the cost is
reasonable and there is a financial incentive for the providers.[43]
What is needed to help accomplish this is innovation in industry. In
the meanwhile, if clinical studies continue to suggest great benefits
for patients pursuing more frequent dialysis at home, and health
care professionals decide to empower their patients with the knowledge of all the options for ESRD care, there may come a critical
point at which patients, dialysis providers, industry and the government come together and we will have a true revival of this excellent
therapy.

References

1. Hegstrom RM, Murray JS, Pendras JP, *et al.* (1961) Hemodialysis in the
   treatment of anemia. *Trans Am Soc Artif Intern Organs* **7**: 136–139.
2. Haviland JW. (1965) Experiences in establishing a community artificial
   kidney center. *Trans Am Clin Clim Assoc* **77**: 125–135.
3. Merrill JP, Schupack E, Cameron. (1964). Hemodialysis in the home.
   JAMA **190**: 468–472.
4. Curtis FK, Cole J, Fellows BJ, *et al.* (1965) Hemodialysis in the home.
   Trans Am Soc Artif Intern Organs **1**: 7–11.
5. Baillod RA, Comty C, Ilahi M. (1965) Overnight haemodialysis in the
   home. In: Kerr DNS (ed.), *Proc Eur Dial Transplant Assoc*, pp. 99–123.
6. Delano BG, Feinroth MV, Feinroth M, Friedman E. (1981) Home and
   medical center hemodialysis: Dollar comparison and payback period.
   JAMA **246**: 230–232.

7. Woods JD, Port FK, Stannard D, *et al.* (1996) Comparison of mortality with home hemodialysis and center hemodialysis: A national study. *Kidney Int* **49**: 1464–1470.

8. Alexander S. (1962) They decide who lives, who dies. *Life Magazine* **Nov. 9**: 102–104.

9. Blagg CR. (1996) A brief history of home hemodialysis. *Adv Ren Replace Ther* **3**: 99–105.

10. Delano BG. (1978) Home hemodialysis. In: Friedman EA (ed.), *Strategy for Renal Failure*, pp. 235–259. John Wiley and Sons, New York.

11. Delano BG, Janes M, Friedman EA. (1981) The paid hemodialysis helper — no panacea. *Proc Clin Dial Transplant Forum* **10**: 138–140.

12. Delano, BG. (1996) Home hemodialysis — major turning points in the past 25 years. *Dial Transplant* **25**: 728–729.

13. US Renal Data System. (2008) USRDS 2008 annual data report. National Institutes of Health, National Institute of Diabetes and Digestive and Kidney Diseases, Bethesda, MD.

14. Popovich RP, Moncrief JW, Nolph KD, *et al.* (1978) Continuous ambulatory peritoneal dialysis. *Ann Intern Med* **88**: 449–456.

15. Bunko M. (2006) Home hemodialysis prevalence varies by country and should be much higher. www.medscape.

16. Delano BG. (1996) Home hemodialysis offers excellent survival. *Adv Ren Replace Ther* **3**: 106–111.

17. Saner E, Kitsch D, Descoeudres C, *et al.* (2005) Outcome of home hemodialysis patients: A case-cohort study. *Nephrol Dial Transplant* **20**: 604–610.

18. Roberts JL. (1976) Analysis and outcome of 1063 patients trained for home hemodialysis. *Kidney Int* **9**: 363–371.

19. Materson, R. (2008) The advantages and disadvantages of home hemodialysis. *Hemodial Int* **12**: S16–S20.

20. Malmstrom RK, Roine RP, Heikkila A, *et al.* (2008) Cost analysis and health-related quality of life of home and self-care satellite haemodialysis. *Nephrol Dial Transplant* **23**: 1990–1996.

21. Howard K, Salkeld, G, White S, *et al.* (2009) The cost-effectiveness of increasing kidney transplantation and home-based dialysis. *Nephrology* Feb. 2 (epublish).

22. Mehrotra R, Marsh D, Vonesh E. (2005) Patient education and access of ESRD patients to renal replacement therapies beyond in-center hemodialysis. *Kidney Int* **68**: 378–390.
23. McLaughlin K, Manns B, Mortis G, *et al.* (2003) Why patients with ESRD do not select self-care dialysis as a treatment option. *Am J Kidney Dis* **41**: 380–385.
24. Nesrallah GE, Suri RS, Moist LM, *et al.* (2008) The International Quotidian Dialysis Registry: Annual Report 2008. *Hemodial Int* **12**: 281–289.
25. Uldall PR, Francoeur R, Ouwendyk M. (1994) Simplified nocturnal home hemodialysis. *J Am Soc Nephrol* **5**: 428–432.
26. Lockridge RS, Pipkin M. (2008) Short and long nightly hemodialysis in the United States. *Hemodial Int* **21**: 48–50.
27. Chan CT, Harvey PJ. (2003) Short term blood pressure, noradrenic and vascular effects of nocturnal home hemodialysis. *Hypertens* **50**: 925–931.
28. Chan CT, Shen XS, Picton P, Floras J. (2008) Nocturnal home hemodialysis improves baroreflex effectiveness index of end stage renal disease patients. *J Hypertens* **26**: 1795–1800.
29. Kundhal K, Pierratos A, Chan CT. (2005) Newer paradigms in renal replacement therapy: Will they alter cardiovascular outcome? *Cardiol Clin* **23**: 385–391.
30. Kooienga L. (2007) Phosphorous balance with daily dialysis. *Semin Dial* **20**: 342–345.
31. Nessim SJ, Jassal SV, Fing SV, Chan CT. (2007) Comparison from conventional to nocturnal hemodialysis improves vitamin D levels. *Kidney Int* **1**: 172–176.
32. Schwartz DI, Pierrates A, Richardson RM, *et al.* (2005) Impact of nocturnal home hemodialysis on anemia management in patients with end-stage renal disease. *Clin Nephrol* **63**: 202–208.
33. Chan CT, Lie PP, Arab S, Jamal N, Messner HA. (2009) Nocturnal hemodialysis improves erythropoietin responsiveness and growth of hematopoietic stem cell. *J Am Soc Nephrol* **20**: 665–671.
34. Unruh ML, Sanders MH, Redline S, *et al.* (2006) Sleep apnea in patients on conventional thrice weekly hemodialysis; comparison with matched controls from the Sleep Heart Health Study. *J Am Soc Nephrol* **17**: 3503–3509.

35. Bugeja AL, Chan CT. (2004) Improvement in lipids profile by nocturnal hemodialysis in patients with end-stage renal disease. *ASAIO J* **17**: 99–103.

36. Manns BJ, Walsh MW, Culleton BF, *et al.* (2009) Nocturnal hemodialysis does not improve overall measures of quality of life compared to conventional hemodialysis. *Kidney Int* **75**: 542–549.

37. Ayus JC, Mizami MR, Achinger SG, *et al.* (2005) The effect of short daily versus conventional hemodialysis on left ventricular hypertrophy and inflammatory markers: A prospective controlled study. *J Am Soc Nephrol* **6**: 2778–2788.

38. Williams AW, Chebrolu SB, Ing TS, *et al.* (2004) Early clinical quality of life and biochemical changes of "daily hemodialysis." *Am J Kidney Dis* **43**: 90–102.

39. Takayuki, H. (2007) Daily versus thrice weekly hemodialysis for phosphorous control. *Nat Clin Pract Nephrol* **3**: 364–365.

40. Suri RS, Nesrallah GE, Mainra G, *et al.* (2006) Daily Hemodialysis: A systematic review. *CJASN* **1**: 33–42.

41. Chazot C, Jean G. (2009) The advantages and challenges of increasing the duration and frequency of maintenance dialysis sessions. *Nat Clin Pract Nephrol* **5**: 34–44.

42. Halpern SD, Berns JS, Israni AK. (2004) Willingness of patients to switch from conventional to daily hemodialysis: Looking before we leap. *Am J Med* **116**: 606–612.

43. Pierratos A. (2008) Daily nocturnal hemodialysis — a paradigm shift worthy of disrupting current dialysis practice. *Nat Clin Pract Nephrol* **4**: 602–603.

44. Shurraw S, Zimmerman D. (2005) Vascular access complications in daily dialysis: A systematic review of the literature. *Minerva Urol Nefrol* **57**: 151–163.

45. Honoken EO, Rauta VM. (2008) What happened in Finland to increase home hemodialysis? *Hemodial Int* **12**: S11–S15.

CHAPTER 5

Hemofiltration

Halim S. Ghali*

Hemofiltration (HF) was first described in 1977 as a means of removing extracellular volume in patients with diuretic-refractory edema. It has many superficial similarities to hemodialysis. In both techniques, access to the circulation is required and blood passes through an extracorporeal circuit that includes either a dialyzer or a hemofilter.

Introduction and Basic Principles

Hemodialysis

Hemodialysis (HD) refers to the transport process by which a solute passively diffuses down its concentration gradient from one fluid compartment (either blood or dialysate) into another. During HD, urea, creatinine, and potassium move from blood to dialysate, while other solutes, such as calcium and bicarbonate, move from dialysate to blood, depending on their relative concentrations. Dialysate flows countercurrent to blood flow through the dialyzer to maximize the concentration gradient between their compartments, thereby maximizing the rate of solute removal. The desired effect is changed plasma concentrations of solutes: reduction in the blood urea nitrogen and plasma creatinine concentration, with concomitant increase in plasma calcium and bicarbonate concentrations. A 4 h HD substitutes

*Clinical Assistant Professor, Renal Division, Department of Medicine; SUNY–Downstate Medical Center. Email: hghali@hotmail.com

for approximately two days of impaired kidney function. HD, however, may cause technique-specific complications that may destabilize critically ill patients, including cardiovascular compromise, hypovolemia and hypotension, dilutional anemia, and a disequilibrium that may include grand mal seizures reflecting the temporary chemical imbalance caused by rapid removal of urea and other nitrogenous wastes.

Patients with advanced illness may be unable to tolerate conventional HD, because they are predisposed to: (a) hypotension due to unstable circulatory dynamics, (b) inability to sustain electrolyte balance, or (c) neuroendocrine, coagulation, and/or fibrinolytic system abnormalities due to extrarenal organ failure. For these patients, continuous renal replacement therapies (CRRTs; see below) may be beneficial, because the rate of change in body compartment chemistry is less marked.

Hemofiltration

Hemofiltration (HF) refers to the use of an induced hydrostatic pressure gradient to effect filtration (or convection) of plasma water across a semipermeable membrane — the hemofilter. The frictional forces between water and solutes (called solvent drag) result in convective transport of small and medium molecular weight solutes (less than 5000 daltons) moving in the same direction as water molecules. Maintenance of plasma volume by infusion of (substitution) fluid is usually required, to prevent excessive fluid removal (see below). The process of HF itself extracts smaller solutes (such as urea and electrolytes) in roughly the same proportion as their plasma concentration. Thus, the plasma concentration of solutes is generally unchanged during HF, in contrast to the usual decrease by HD. Administration of substitution fluid does, by dilution, lower the plasma concentrations of all solutes (including urea and creatinine) not present in the substitution fluid. The patient's blood is pumped through a filtration circuit to a semipermeable filter, where solutes and water are removed. After leaving the hemofilter, substitution fluid is added and blood is returned to the patient. As in HD, in HF solutes traverse a semipermeable membrane, though in HF solute movement is governed by convection rather than by diffusion. HF does not employ a dialysate. Instead, positive hydrostatic pressure drives water and solutes across the filter membrane from the blood compartment to the filtrate compartment, from which it is drained. The small and large solutes are dragged through membrane pores at a similar rate by water flow governed by hydrostatic pressure. In HF, convection overcomes the reduced removal rate of larger solutes (due to their slow speed of diffusion) seen in HD. There are various types of HF, some of which depend purely on the systolic blood pressure of the patient as a driving force and some depend on the introduction of a pump to ensure driving pressure (see below).

Hemodiafiltration

HF can be used in combination with HD, when it is known as hemodi-afiltration (HDF). In HDF, solute extraction is effected approximately 75% by diffusion and 25% or more by convection (filtration).

As generally practiced, in HDF blood is pumped through a compartment of a high flux dialyzer, and subjected to a high rate of ultrafiltration to maximize movement of water and solutes from blood to dialysate, after which blood volume is maintained by infusion of a substitution fluid directly into the postdialyzer blood line. However, dialysis solution is also run through the dialysate compartment of the dialyzer. The combination of dialysis (diffusion-based solute removal) and filtration (convection-based solute and water removal) treatments is theoretically useful, because it results in a balanced extraction of both high and low molecular weight solutes.

Substitution fluid

Isotonic replacement fluid is added to the blood line before it is returned to the patient. This replacement fluid is infused directly into the blood line of the extracorporeal circuit. It can be added either pre- or postfilter (pre- or postdilution; see below).

Replacement HF fluid usually contains lactate or acetate as a bicarbonate-generating base, or bicarbonate itself. Administration of lactate must be restricted in patients with lactic acidosis or severe liver disease, who may be unable to effect conversion of lactate to bicarbonate. For such patients a bicarbonate base must be used.

HF and HDF can be administered intermittently or continuously. Continuous treatment is usually accomplished in an intensive care unit setting.

Intermittent Modes of Therapy: On-Line Intermittent Hemodialysis, Hemofiltration and Hemodiafiltration

Extracorporeal intermittent treatment of patients in renal failure or suffering fluid and/or solute abnormalities may be accomplished with either dialysis (diffusion-based solute removal) or filtration (convection-based solute and water removal) treatments that operate in an intermittent mode. Either treatment can be delivered in outpatient dialysis units, in a regimen applied three or more times a week, usually 3–5 h per treatment. With both on-line intermittent hemofiltration (IHF) and on-line intermittent hemodiafiltration (IHDF), substitution fluid is prepared on-line from a dialysis solution by running dialysis solution through a set of two membranes to purify it before its infusion directly into the blood line. There is a current controversy about whether on-line IHDF gives superior results when compared with on-line intermittent HD in an outpatient setting. In Europe, several observational studies compared outcomes in patients treated with HD and IHDF, "suggesting" a lower mortality rate and other favorable outcomes in patients in the IHDF group. No randomized, prospective controlled clinical trials have been reported, limiting the application of these studies. Another limitation of the comparisons of HD and IHDF is that while dialysis was performed using low flux (small pore) membranes, IHDF employed a high flux membrane, permitting the combination of convective transport (filtration) with dialysis.

In the United States, regulatory agencies have not yet approved on-line creation of substitution fluid because of concerns about its purity. For this reason, HDF is almost never used in an outpatient setting in the United States. Routine use of currently available sterile, prepackaged substitution fluid is cost-prohibitive. A recent Cochrane database review of available trials could not find a definite benefit of either IHF or IHDF versus intermittent HD in terms of outcomes. The United States Renal Data System Annual Data Report for 2008 does not mention HF in any of its varieties and hence does not permit comparison of survival attributed to this technique.

Continuous Renal Replacement Therapies: Continuous Hemofiltration and Hemodiafiltration

Continuous renal replacement therapies (CRRTs) involve either dialysis (diffusion-based solute removal) or filtration (convection-based solute and water removal) treatments that operate in a continuous mode. Variations of CRRT can extend the treatment duration to 12–24 h, especially during daytime periods of full staffing. The longer duration of CRRT makes it quite different from conventional intermittent therapies, in which each treatment lasts 4–6 h or less. A major advantage attributed to continuous therapy is a slower rate of solute or fluid removal per unit of time. Thus, CRRT is thought to be generally better-tolerated than conventional therapy, since many of the complications of intermittent therapies are related to the rapid rate of solute and fluid loss with resultant hypotensive episodes. CRRT has mainly been utilized in critical care and intensive care units.

CRRT has been classified into: (1) continuous hemofiltration (CHF), for removal of water, body waste, and pathogenic substances through filtration; (2) continuous hemodialysis (CHD), for removal of water, body waste, and pathogenic substances through diffusion using dialysate; and (3) continuous hemodiafiltration (CHDF), for removal of water, body waste, and pathogenic substances through both filtration and diffusion using dialysate.

CRRT techniques initially utilized arteriovenous extracorporeal circuits in which blood flow was driven by the gradient between the mean arterial pressure and venous pressure. Continuous venovenous hemofiltration (CVVH) and continuous venovenous hemodialysis (CVVHD) were developed in the mid-1980s as alternatives to continuous arteriovenous hemofiltration (CAVH) and continuous arteriovenous hemodialysis (CAVHD). The use of a pump-driven venovenous circuit in venovenous CRRT permits blood flows that are both higher and more constant than that provided by an arteriovenous circuit. In addition, since there is no need for a large bore arterial catheter, the associated risks of arterial thrombosis and arterial bleeding are eliminated.

CRRTs are proposed as indicated in patients with severe acute pancreatitis, fulminant hepatitis, postoperative liver failure, multiple organ failure, cardiovascular disease, and severe renal failure.

CHF has been used exclusively in intensive care settings, almost always restricted to acute renal failure. When it is applied as a slow continuous therapy, the terms "slow extended hemofiltration" (SLEF; over 8–12 h) and "slow continuous ultrafiltration" (SCUF; over 12–24 h) have been used. HD and HDF are also widely used in this fashion: CHD, slow extended hemodiafiltration (SLEHDF) and CHDF.

In the United States, the substitution fluid used in CHF or CHDF is commercially prepared, prepackaged, and sterile (or sometimes it is prepared in the local hospital pharmacy), avoiding regulatory issues of on-line creation of replacement fluid from dialysis solution.

With slow continuous therapies, blood flow rates ranging from 100 to 200 ml/min are attained with a blood pump via a vascular access through a central venous catheter. Current thought precludes use of conventional hemodialysis vascular access (arteriovenous fistulae or grafts) for slow continuous therapies, because prolonged presence of access needles could damage the access.

CRRT access characteristics — venovenous or arteriovenous

Different modalities are categorized according to the required access characteristics. Arteriovenous (AV) access refers to the use of an arterial catheter that allows blood to flow into the extracorporeal circuit by virtue of the systemic blood pressure. A venous catheter is placed for return. AV therapies have the advantage of blood flow and filtration determined by blood pressure. This offers a theoretical advantage of fewer hypotensive episodes. AV circuitry is simple to rapidly set up and requires a low volume extracorporeal system with low resistance, obviating the need for expensive and complex extracorporeal pumps and circuits.

But AV therapies are unable to attain the higher volumes of ultrafiltration required for consistent metabolic control. Blood flow may be unreliable in patients who are hypotensive or who have severe peripheral vascular disease. Also, AV therapies require arterial puncture with a large bore (femoral) artery catheter, with an attendant risk of arterial embolization. The risk of vascular complications has been estimated to be up to 10%. For these reasons AV therapy modalities are seldom used.

Venovenous (VV) access is an alternative modality in which both catheters or one dual lumen catheter is placed in veins. An extracorporeal blood pump is required to circulate blood through the extracorporeal circuit. VV access does not require arterial access, involves less systemic anticoagulation, uses only one dual lumen catheter, and has faster and more reliable blood flow than arterial access. A key disadvantage of VV regimens is the requirement for an extracorporeal blood pump. However, the availability of inexpensive, reliable double lumen venous catheters is stimulating further exploration of VV modalities.

Anticoagulation during CRRT

In CRRT modalities, clotting of the extracorporeal system is the most common technical problem and anticoagulation is generally required to maintain system patency.

Heparin

Heparin is the most commonly utilized anticoagulant. Typically, a bolus dose of 1000–2000 units of heparin is administered into the inflow ("arterial") limb of the extracorporeal circuit, followed by a continuous infusion of 300–500 units per hour. Therapy may be monitored by following the partial thromboplastin time in the outflow ("venous") limb; the heparin dose should be titrated to maintain a value of 1.5–2.0 times control. Larger doses of heparin may be required in patients with recurrent system clotting. Its discontinuation may be necessary in the setting of clinical bleeding or if severe thrombocytopenia develops.

Citrate

Regional citrate anticoagulation has been widely used as an alternative to heparin in all modalities of CRRT. During citrate anticoagulation, sodium citrate is infused into the inflow ("arterial") limb of the extracorporeal circuit, chelating calcium and thereby inhibiting clotting. Intravenous calcium must be infused systemically to maintain a normal ionized serum calcium concentration. The use of citrate anticoagulation may require modification of the dialysate composition.

Since citrate provides an alkali load, buffers (e.g. bicarbonate, lactate) may need to be reduced in concentration or deleted from the dialysate and replacement fluids. The dialysate and replacement fluids should also be calcium-free to prevent reversal of the citrate effect in the extracorporeal circuit. If a hypertonic citrate solution is utilized, the sodium concentration in the dialysate and/or replacement fluids will need to be reduced so as to prevent the development of hypernatremia.

Selection of anticoagulation

Selection of the anticoagulation method is not evidence-based and has generally been dictated by local practice. Each method has its inherent risks:

- Heparin-induced thrombocytopenia with heparin anticoagulation;
- Metabolic alkalosis and hypocalcemia from citrate toxicity with citrate anticoagulation.

Several studies have suggested more prolonged filter patency using citrate anticoagulation. However, this benefit needs to be balanced against the increased costs associated with citrate anticoagulation.

Forms of continuous renal replacement therapies

Slow extended hemofiltration

In slow extended hemofiltration (SLEF), or slow continuous ultrafiltration (SCUF), the extracorporeal system is simplified to include a blood system hooked in line with a high efficiency or high flux membrane. As blood passes through the membrane, plasma water and solutes pass through it to allow formation of an ultrafiltrate, which is discarded. No replacement fluids or dialysate fluids are required. Although SLEF is a purely convective modality, the ultrafiltrate volume is limited to inputs plus desired losses and hence there is not enough volume to control azotemia or significant metabolic disorders. This regimen has been applied to patients with substantive residual renal function but high volumes of input and/or significant fluid overload with a "relative" oliguria. SLEF, or SCUF, is strictly a dehydrating procedure with no aim of substantially removing solute. Access can be AV or VV.

SLEF has mainly been utilized when fluid removal goals are modest. CRRT modalities designed for fluid and metabolic control require higher volumes of ultrafiltrate and hence require replacement fluid, dialysate fluid, or a combination of the two, as described below.

Continuous venovenous hemofiltration

Continuous venovenous hemofiltration (CVVH) is an extracorporeal circuit with a double lumen venous catheter hooked to an extracorporeal system with a blood pump, a high efficiency or high flux dialysis membrane, and replacement fluid (see Fig. 1). As in SLEF, pure convection produces an ultrafiltrate — which is,

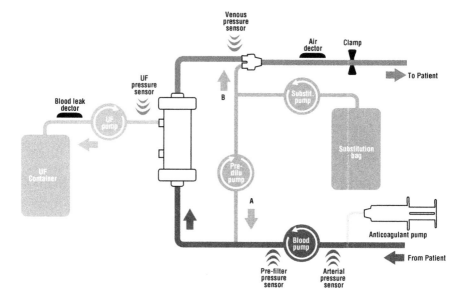

Fig. 1. CVVH substitution fluid is predilution (A) or postdilution (B).

however, generated in much greater volume. The patient's plasma volume and metabolic improvements are maintained by addition of replacement fluid to the circuit. Replacement fluid can be added pre- or postdilution (pre- or postfilter). Prefilter replacement carries a benefit of less hemoconcentration within the dialysis membrane but decreases clearances by up to 15%. Postfilter replacement maintains efficiency of the circuit but may be associated with an increased risk of thrombosis of the extracorporeal circuit.

Continuous arteriovenous hemofiltration

Continuous arteriovenous hemofiltration (CAVH) uses an AV access to remove fluid and solutes by convection. Its per-hour efficiency of solute extraction is generally low, as no diffusion occurs. Thus, if employed as a renal replacement therapy, 24 h/day application or addition of enhancing techniques is required.

Continuous venovenous hemodialysis

Continuous venovenous hemodialysis (CVVHD) is an extracorporeal therapy in which a double lumen venous catheter is hooked to an extracorporeal system utilizing a blood pump, a high efficiency or high flux dialysis membrane, and dialysate fluid. As in intermittent HD, the dialysate runs countercurrent to the blood pathway. Volume status and metabolic improvements are maintained by addition of pre- or postfilter replacement fluid to the circuit.

While CVVHD is considered a diffusive therapy, convection also occurs due to both the high permeability of the membrane and back-filtration. The amount of back-filtration and convective clearance probably varies according to the specific membrane employed, though this component of therapy has not been studied to date.

Continuous arteriovenous hemodialysis

Continuous arteriovenous hemodialysis (CAVHD) is similar to CAVH, with the addition of continuous perfusion of dialysate through the hemofilter countercurrent to the direction of blood flow, most commonly at a rate of 1–2 L per hour. The technical requirements for satisfactory performance of CAVHD are similar to those for CAVH. With CAVHD, blood flow through the extracorporeal circuit is driven by the gradient between mean systemic arterial and venous pressures. Ultrafiltration is achieved by use of HF membranes with high hydraulic permeability. The presence of dialysate in CAVHD augments total solute removal by adding diffusive solute clearance to the convective solute transport of CAVH. Fluid removal is slower than with CAVH alone, but a greater reduction in solute concentration is achieved. CAVHD was developed to improve solute clearances obtainable with CAVH. Although the latter provides excellent volume control, solute clearances are frequently insufficient to provide satisfactory control of azotemia, particularly in hypercatabolic patients. Ultrafiltration is limited to the rate at which net fluid removal is desired and no intravenous fluid replacement is required.

Continuous venovenous hemodiafiltration

Continuous venovenous hemodiafiltration (CVVHDF) consists of an extracorporeal circuit with a double lumen venous catheter hooked to an extracorporeal system with a blood pump, a high efficiency or high flux dialysis membrane, and both replacement and dialysate fluid (see Fig. 2). CVVHDF combines diffusive and convective solute transport — a combination that increases solute clearance determined by both diffusive and convective forces. Its efficacy is improved for higher molecular weight solutes (small proteins, mediators, etc.), as well as for small molecular weight substances (urea, creatinine, electrolytes, and buffer base). HDF combines the advantages of HF and HD by performing the two procedures in parallel. It combines the solute removal capabilities of HF and HD. As with CVVH, a large ultrafiltrate volume is generated across a membrane with high

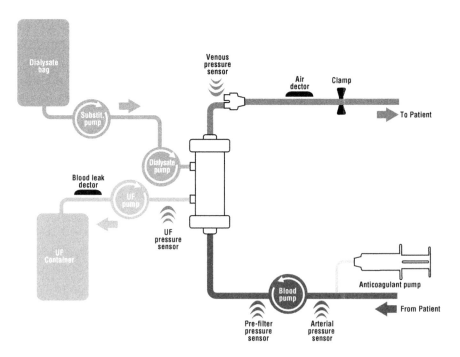

Fig. 2.   CVVHDF substitution fluid here is postdilution.

hydraulic permeability. Replacement fluid is infused into the extra-corporeal circuit, either before (predilution) or after (postdilution) the hemodiafilter replacing the volume of ultrafiltrate that is in excess of the desired net negative fluid removal. In addition, as in CVVHD, dialysate is perfused through the hemodiafilter, countercurrent to the direction of blood flow.

Continuous arteriovenous hemodiafiltration

Continuous arteriovenous hemodiafiltration (CAVHDF) is similar to CAVHD except that ultrafiltration is allowed at a rate beyond that necessary for re-establishing euvolemia. From the viewpoint of solute removal, CAVHDF combines removal of small solutes by diffusion with removal of large solutes by convection. Because the volume of fluid ultrafiltered is so large, replacement fluid must be given to maintain euvolemia.

Choice of therapy

Whether any CRRT offers either survival or other benefits when compared with currently utilized intermittent renal replacement therapies is an unresolved issue. Those head-to-head comparisons that have been reported have not established superiority for continuous therapy. The choice of modality is dependent upon several factors, including availability, the expertise of the clinician, hemodynamic stability, vascular access, and whether the primary need is for fluid and/or solute removal. This last factor is often an important determinant, since each of these procedures is associated with a different rate of solute and water removal.

Examples

SLEF (or SCUF), CAVH, or CVVH can be used if fluid removal is the primary goal. VV access is generally preferred because of its more predictable blood flow rate. However, AV access can be used if blood pumps are not available.

CAVHDF and CVVHDF are more effective than CAVH or CVVH in the highly catabolic patient with a large small solute load. CAVHDF and CVVHDF combine the convective solute removal of continuous hemofiltration (CAVH and CVVH) with the diffusive solute removal of continuous hemodialysis (CAVHD and CVVHD).

Specific indications for CRRT

Acute renal failure

Either form of CRRT can be used in management of acute renal failure. By combining convective and diffusive solute clearance, CAVHDF and CVVHDF provide augmented solute clearance at any given dialysate flow rate as compared with both CAVHD and CVVHD. Improved clearance of "middle" molecular weight substances is a theoretical (not clinically proven) benefit of convective therapy. This benefit is balanced by the increased technical complexity and nursing effort necessitated by the continuous monitoring and replacement of large volumes of ultrafiltrate required with CAVHDF and CVVHDF. In management of acute renal failure, CAVHD has largely been supplanted by CVVHD. Unlike CAVHD, blood flow with CVVHD does not depend upon mean arterial pressure since a blood pump is utilized, thereby providing a higher and more constant blood flow. In addition, the VVs system avoids risks associated with prolonged, large bore arterial catheters. However, the use of a VVs system entails increased technological complexity, including blood pumps, air detectors, and pressure monitors.

Contrast-media-induced nephropathy

Although further studies are needed, there are some advocates who suggest that HF is an effective means of reducing the risk of contrast-media-induced nephropathy in patients with chronic kidney disease undergoing intravenous-contrast-involved-procedures. Pre-HF has been suggested to obtain the full clinical benefit as, among the different mechanisms possibly involved, high-volume controlled hydration before contrast media exposure may play a major role.

Septic shock

One of the forms of HDF, CAVHDF or CVVHDF with its convective removal of larger solutes, may be desirable in the patient with sepsis in whom an ancillary goal is the removal of inflammatory mediators. The use of high volume, continuous forms of HDF (either continuous AV or VV) benefits the hemodynamic course and outcome in patients with intractable circulatory failure resulting from septic shock. This form of management is expensive, requires defined expertise, and may be associated with metabolic and coagulation abnormalities. Further studies are needed to determine if this mode of therapy improves outcome in septic patients. Its use should probably be limited to patients with renal indications for HDF.

Conclusions

Continuous hemofiltration delivered in several technical variations is a highly effective system for replacement of renal function, especially in patients with acute renal failure. Due to its continuous control of the rate of solute and water extraction, patients treated by HF rarely suffer unwanted alteration of extracellular volume, even following administration of large volumes of fluid, for nutritional or other purposes. HF applied to patients in acute renal failure is a safe renal replacement therapy that may reduce overall morbidity as injured kidneys recover. It must be emphasized that in terms of evidence-based medicine, in patients with renal failure who are subjected to renal replacement therapy, benefits for any application of HF over HD or for continuous over intermittent treatments are unproven. Even the simplest form of HD employing prepackaged dialysate flowing through disposable cartridges and tubing is too expensive for the vast majority of the world — a reality meaning that there is little room for complex continuous regimens that are labor- and intensive-care-unit-dependent.

References

1. Canaud B, Bragg-Gresham JL, Marshall MR, Desmeules S, Gillespie BW, Depner T, Klassen P, Port FK. (2006) Mortality risk for patients receiving IHDF versus hemodialysis: European results from the DOPPS. *Kidney Int* **69**(11): 2087–2093.

2. Rabindranath KS, Strippoli GF, Daly C, Roderick PJ, Wallace S, MacLeod AM. (2006) Hemodiafiltration, hemofiltration and hemodialysis for end-stage kidney disease. *Cochrane Database Syst Rev* **4**: CD006258.

3. Manns M, Sigler MH, Teehan BP. (1998) Continuous renal replacement therapies: An update. *Am J Kidney Dis* **32**: 185.

4. Kanagasundaram NS, Paganini EP. (1999) Critical care dialysis — a Gordian knot (but is untying the right approach?). *Nephrol Dial Transplant* **14**: 2590.

5. Ronco C, Bellomo R, Kellum JA. (2002) Continuous renal replacement therapy: Opinions and evidence. *Adv Ren Replace Ther* **9**: 229.

6. Mehta RL. (2005) Continuous renal replacement therapy in the critically ill patient. *Kidney Int* **67**: 781.

7. McCarthy JT, Moran J, Posen G, Leypoldt JK. (2003) A time for rediscovery: Chronic hemofiltration for end-stage renal disease. *Semin Dial* **16**: 199.

8. Palevsky PM. (2006) Dialysis modality and dosing strategy in acute renal failure. *Semin Dial* **19**: 165.

9. Forni LG, Hilton PJ. (1997) Continuous hemofiltration in the treatment of acute renal failure. *N Eng J Med* **336**: 1303–1309.

CHAPTER 6

Self-Care In-Center Hemodialysis

*Susan H. Bray**

The purpose of this chapter is to discuss the modality of hemodialysis performed by the patient in the hemodialysis center. This is self-care in-center hemodialysis (SCICHD), a modality which allows the patient to move from a level of near-total dependency to independence. Patient education allows the patient to gain control over the hemodialysis procedure. SCICHD can be performed in the home once the patient is trained in the modality or the patient may continue to perform the modality in the outpatient center. SCICHD is empowering and gives control to patients who have become end-stage.[1–3]

The process of beginning a dialysis regimen has been disempowering for many patients, who feel victimized and helpless due to the loss of their vital kidney function and the need to be kept alive by artificial means. Education helps to overcome the sense of helplessness and allows patients to return to an active lifestyle, with improved physical and emotional well-being.

In the mid-1980s, Morton and Mears looked at self-care delivery of hemodialysis and concluded that healthcare quality of life, in terms of functional status and well-being, was statistically better in patients trained for self-care hemodialysis.[4] The patients scored higher than the staff-assisted patients in psychosocial measures in health-related quality of life issues. These higher scores persisted over time. Their physiological measurements remained similar to the

*Clinical Associate Professor, College of Medicine, Drexel University, Philadelphia, Pennsylvania, USA. Email: sjhbray@comcast.net

measurements of patients who were tightly watched in a standard staff-assisted center. The self-care group included diabetic patients and patients with ischemic heart disease, as well as peripheral vascular disease, and were not a statistically different group with regard to co-morbid diseases than the maintenance dialysis group. In spite of similar co-morbid conditions, the patients did very well in the self-care unit with regard to scores on health related quality of life issues. There was no significant difference in creatinine, albumin, hemoglobin, or Kt/V. The authors theorize that the *perception* of improved energy and psychosocial well-being may well be the result of the autonomy and return of a sense of control associated with the self-care process. Self-care provided, from the patient's perspective, a clearer understanding of the process of hemodialysis and of the function of the kidneys prior to renal failure, and allowed the patients to adapt to their illness and to reassert their autonomy.[2,5] Other studies examining patient control have found that a sense of control over health and life in general contributes to psychosocial well-being.[6–8]

Programming to enhance patient knowledge, physical and vocational functioning, and emotional well-being in dialysis has been linked to reduced staff turnover and improved patient outcomes.[9,11,13] There are, however, barriers to patient empowerment.[11,12,18] Several of the key reasons for the lack of patient empowerment include the following:[1,7,11]

- *Paternalism.* An acute disease model is used in providing dialysis care in general, and in this model professionals are the knowledgeable experts and the patient is a "patient." The model, however, is not appropriate for chronic disease, because the goal of treatment is not necessarily *cure*, but rather *adjustment* — adjustment to day-to-day symptom management. Patients who survive for long periods of time (decades) self-manage independently and consult with their care teams as equals. Changing over to an empowering chronic disease model requires a shift in staff attitude and behavior, which in the long run improves staff satisfaction because the staff is more challenged to provide education to patients and to be involved in their development and progression toward self-management.

- *Lack of health literacy.* Patients who are new to dialysis rarely are knowledgeable about what it involves. For many of them, the learning curve is quite steep because of pre-existing ignorance about kidney disease and how it is treated.
- *Patient fear and denial.* New patients may also be quite terrified, angry, depressed, and overwhelmed. Their fear and denial may lead staff to believe that the patients do not want to learn or do not want a role in their care. It is very easy for patients in this frame of mind to become passive, dependent, and to have the impression that only a professional can administer a dialysis treatment.
- *Physician or staff reticence.* Staff or physicians may refuse to allow patients to engage in self-management. This is due to a multiplicity of concerns, the greatest probably being that of litigation. It appears to be an unfounded concern.
- *Lack of availability of the modality.* Self-care dialysis training is not widely available, and patients often have no idea that the modality even exists. Why facilities and nephrologists and nephrology teams have failed to teach the patients about the availability of the modality, and also failed to provide the modality, is an unanswered question. In a large national study on this issue, only about 25% of patients reported having been told about peritoneal dialysis or home hemodialysis, and even fewer about the possibility of self-care in-center dialysis.
- *Physician apathy.* It does take extra effort and a change in mindset to enable patients, through education, to become more knowledgeable and to gain some control over their dialysis regimens. This may be the barrier to the successful development of a self-care in-center hemodialysis training program. Having a successful program demands complete commitment to that modality from the staff and the physician.
- *Economic constraints.* These exist because it does take staff a longer time to train patients than to just sit them down and begin

dialysis; however, when the patients are trained, the fact that they have excellent longevity and quality of life and fewer hospitalizations should cost the system less over time.

- *Impaired vision and/or impaired dexterity.* These can be overcome by special teaching methods and by having staff offer assistance to patients with physical limitations, while still encouraging them to be involved as much as possible in their dialysis.
- *Concern for increased risk of errors by patients.* This risk is minimized as patients become educated about the dialytic process. They are considerably more careful with their dialysis treatments because they realize the importance of doing the procedure correctly.
- *Basic laziness of human beings.* If a patient initiates staff-assisted hemodialysis, and then is expected to gradually move into the modality of self-care in-center hemodialysis, he or she is often hesitant about learning to perform the treatment. He/she becomes a "patient" and will remain in a dependent relationship with staff instead of developing independence through education.

Table 1.   Barriers to SCICHD

(1) Physician apathy
(2) Physician paternalism
(3) Economic uncertainties
(4) Legal concerns
(5) Lack of physician/staff commitment
(6) Economic constraints
(7) Impaired vision/dexterity
(8) Fear of increased patient self-responsibility
(9) Patient reticence
(10) Concern over possible increased risk of error by the patient/staff
(11) Patient lack of knowledge about the existence of the modality
(12) Limited availability of self-care training facilities
(13) Fear of technical aspects of hemodialysis and venipuncture
(14) Patient/staff inertia

How do facilities decide to go about empowering patients? A major step is to offer predialysis education in the chronic kidney disease (CKD) clinic setting. This does not routinely happen. However, simply realizing how vital it is for patients to develop control is the first step. No one accidentally or passively survives for decades on dialysis. In a CKD setting, the job of dialysis professionals is not only to provide care but also to prepare patients to manage their own care, both inside the dialysis facility and outside the facility. Preparing the patients for SCICHD is empowering for the staff as well as for the patients, since it includes education for self-management rather than just providing dialysis care to patients.

Another step in empowering patients to have control over their dialysis is to demystify the process of dialysis and to create an expectation that patients will, in fact, be involved in their own care.[6,13,14] This expectation must be obvious to the patient from the very first day of dialysis, and preferably, from well before the first day of dialysis. The ideal place for the education to begin is the CKD clinic setting. This predialysis education will serve to minimize stress and to help the patient make educated choices regarding the treatment modality, the need to learn how to deal with emotionally sensitive aspects of living with renal failure, death of peers, and the need to live meaningfully within the constraints imposed by the treatment. Ongoing education of self-care patients might include the following:[1,3,7,8,15]

- Integration of nutritional education;
- Counseling and psychosocial support for all self-care kidney patients in the facility;
- Periodic refresher courses on the technical and procedural developments affecting the hemodialysis treatment;
- Peer group counseling and one-on-one peer communication.

More controlled intradialytic fluid weight gains occur. Since the patients are taught to self-cannulate, observational data reveal fewer access problems and longer survival of dialysis grafts and fistulae. Interestingly, there has been no documented increase in access infection as compared with in-center staff-assisted hemodialysis-related access infection. Observational data also show far fewer episodes of cramping and hypotension than in staff-assisted in-center hemodialysis.[16]

When considering patients for the SCICHD facility training program, there are a few criteria that need to be followed. The first and most important one is the patient's desire to learn the modality. The patient should be medically stable and have at least some vision and dexterity. A functioning access is a requirement. The patient must agree to adhere to the expectations of the program, which include taking medications, being punctual for treatment, and performing the dialysis procedure precisely.[1,17,18]

SCICHD as a modality can well serve as a bridge to home hemodialysis, both in the United States and in developing countries, where the patient may have very long distances to travel in order to get to an outpatient facility. Self-care hemodialysis can be utilized in the standard three-times-a-week fashion, or can be utilized nightly or for short, daily hemodialysis either in-center or at home and can be well utilized in satellite centers with limited dialysis staff, especially in the rural areas of the United States and in developing countries.[6,19,20] In some areas, there is no health care professional on site and patients perform their treatments without supervision. Only medically stable patients are allowed into these satellite facilities. If they become ill or generally unstable they are transferred to a more traditional facility.[21]

There is little recent data specifically addressing SCICHD. Seminal work, publication, and encouragement of the modality was done by Stanley Shaldon in France in the 1960s, at which time he

Table 2.   Patient Selection Criteria

(1) Patient desire to learn
(2) Stable medical condition
(3) Functioning access
(4) Basic manual dexterity
(5) Some vision
(6) Adherence to expectations of the program

had excellent results with his patients, proving that dialysis can be safely performed outside of the hospital setting by the patient, even in the home. This was hugely important to the further development of chronic dialysis as all patients were dialyzed in hospital at that time.[3,20,22]

There is a reduced mortality rate in the self-care population: 7–9% as compared with the national death rate of 23%. There is a definite decrease in hospitalization rates and lengths of stay, with the average stay of a US dialysis patient being 17 days and that of the self-care patient being an average of 9 days per year. It has been found that there is a slight decrease in the erythropoietin-stimulating agent dose and the reasons for this are not scientifically clear, but may reflect a good response to regular treatment and excellent dialysis adequacy.[23] Patients have better phosphate control as a direct result of their education and adherence to medications.[12,15]

Quality of life scores are improved over those of the staff-assisted hemodialysis patients and are comparable to those of home hemodialysis patients and transplant patients.[4,8,10,24] Controlled studies are needed which compare the outcomes of SCICHD to those of standard, staff-assisted in-center dialysis and of home hemodialysis. There are, over time, fewer costs associated with this modality.[14,19,23,25] It is possible to have fewer staff available on site and those who are there are involved in the teaching of new patients and re-education of returning patients, as well as oversight of individual patients' activities in performing their dialysis. It is a definite change in the mindset of the health care professionals from that of "nurturing and doing" to that of educating and encouraging independence.[18]

Staff is affected by the presence of this modality. There can be decreased numbers as mentioned, but also a definite change in the activities of the staff. Their activities are geared much more towards education of the patient about the technical and medical aspects of dialysis, basic renal function and dysfunction, and less devoted to the more rote provision of the dialysis procedure. The staff members become educators of new staff about the philosophy of self-care and thereby of returning control to patients via this modality. The staff members note decreased drudgery because of the ever-changing challenges involved in the education process.[1,17]

Improved financial considerations can be expected via several mechanisms. Lower hospitalization rates and shorter lengths of stay cost the system less, and allow improved income to the dialysis facility since the patients are not off-site, being dialyzed in the hospital. Death rates are lower and there is a much smaller number of missed dialyses, which by itself is associated with improved survival. With improved adherence, which is a direct result of the education of the patient, the patient becomes more stable, with less nursing acuity demanded. There is a lower staff turnover due to better job satisfaction, and more clinically stable treatments, and thus less use of special expensive drugs for treatment of unstable patients.[18,19,23,25]

What is the future picture for SCICHD? Hopefully, it will be recognized by CMS and carriers as a superior modality, and be better reimbursed. There will be financial incentives for facilities to develop and manage self-care hemodialysis programs. Development of regional centers for self-care training is one possibility, using self-care training as a bridge to dialysis therapy at home. The development of regional centers in other countries might be envisioned, with the application of SCICHD in less populated areas having decreased availability of trained dialysis staff. More scientific data is needed to support the medical superiority of SCICHD to other in-center modalities. The utilization of SCICHD and all possible applications, including nocturnal, daily, three-times-a-week, and

Table 3.   Clinical Advantages

(1) Lower hospitalization rates
(2) Lower mortality
(3) Better QoL scores
(4) Return to work/school
(5) Smaller number of missed treatments
(6) Better adherence
(7) Return of sense of control

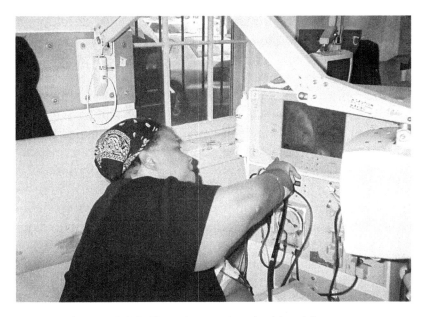

Fig. 1. SCICHD patient setting the blood flow rate.

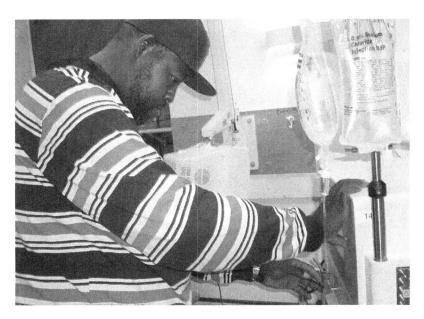

Fig. 2. SCICHD patient preparing the dialyzer.

every other day, will be a reality in the future. New developments in technology which is simpler to use, more efficient, and has better safety features will facilitate self-care, both in-center and at home. There will be standards of care developed for SCICHD. The return to employment, or to education by all possible patients, will be celebrated and strongly encouraged. Patients will have excellent nutrition, an improved body mass index, and normalization of their laboratory studies. There will be appropriate health care insurance for the modality, so that there will be no insurance barrier towards providing it. The patients should come to experience improved exercise tolerance, and normalization of blood pressure, hematocrit, and bone mineral metabolism. Psychosocial improvements will be observed, including improved quality of life scores. All possible patients should be on the active transplant list in the future. Also in the future, the self-care patients can and will serve as mentors or teachers to incoming patients and will assist in the training

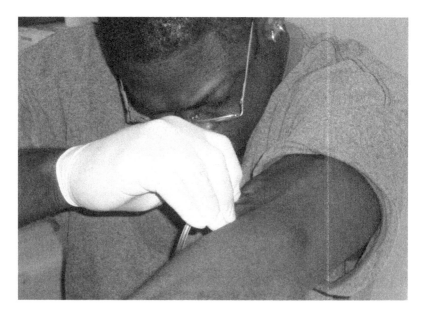

Fig. 3. 23-year-old type I diabetic patient on hemodialysis for 5 months inserting hemodialysis needles after instruction.

of the new patients. CKD clinics with modality education curricula will be the standard of care for CKD patients progressing towards stage V. Third World countries will be able to more efficiently offer dialysis as a self-care modality leading to home dialysis. The health-related quality of life scores will be measured as an outcome of self-care hemodialysis, and can be compared to outcomes in maintenance dialysis. Regional training centers for home and in-center self-care will be developed to conserve resources and maximize efficiency.[19,22]

In conclusion, self-care in-center hemodialysis is an excellent modality for patients to utilize. It can be performed in the standard three-times-a-week fashion, or more frequently if the center is committed to providing more frequent dialysis, or, as a natural outcome, in the home thrice weekly or daily/nightly. Patients are psychologically healthier, because they have regained control, in a huge way, over their medical condition (ESRD), including the machine on which their lives depend. They become and/or remain physically healthier, emotionally move contended, and survive longer and better. SCICHD can be used either as a bridge to home dialysis or as the in-center regimen of choice.

References

1. Bray S. (2006) Returning control to ESRD patients through self-care in-center hemodialysis. *KTimes* **2**: 1–5.
2. Lefcourt H. (1973) The function of the illusion of control and freedom. *Am Psychol* **28**: 417–425.
3. Bray SH, Hood SS. (1983) Nutrition therapy using *ad libitum* diet and protein encouragement in chronic hemodialysis therapy. *CRN Q* **7**: 17–18.
4. Bray S, Jones E. (1986) In-center self-care hemodialysis (SCICHD) is associated with high patient rehabilitation rates (*abstract*). *Am Soc Nephrol.*
5. Bremer B, McCauley C, Wrona R, Johnson J. (1989) Quality of life in end-stage renal disease: A reexamination. *Am J Kidney Dis* **13**: 200–209.
6. Latham C. (1998) Is there data to support the concept that educated, empowered patients have better outcomes? *J Am Soc Nephrol* **9**: S141–S144.

7. Devins G, Benik T, *et al.* (1984) The emotional impact of end-stage renal disease: Importance of patients' perceptions of intrusiveness and control. *Int J Psy Med* **13**(4): 327–343.

8. Bray S. (2003) Does self-care dialysis improve quality of life for ESRD patients? *Contemp Dial Nephrol* **24**: 2–5.

9. Bray S. (1993) A primer for initiating a self-care dialysis program. iKidney.com.

10. Greenfield S, Kaplan S. (1985) Expanding patient involvement in care: Effects on patient outcomes. *Ann Intern Med* **102**: 520–528.

11. Schatell D, Witten B, *et al.* (2005) Dialysis patient empowerment: What, why and how. *Nephrol News Issues*, 37–39, Aug.

12. Kaplan DeNour A, Czaczkes J. (1976) The influence of patients' personality on adjustment to chronic dialysis. *J Ner Ment Dis* **162**(5): 323–333.

13. Dobby AS. (1992) Self-care hemodialysis training and autonomy: The patients' perspective. *CAANT* **17**: 2–4.

14. Newmann J. (1994) Education and patient empowerment. *Nephrol News Issues* 22–27.

15. Bray S. (2004) Tips on how to initiate self-care hemodialysis in your facility. *Nephrol Incite* **15**.

16. Shaldon S, *et al.* (1963) *Br Med J* **1**: 1717–1718.

17. Easton KL. (1993) Defining the concept of self-care. *Rehabil Nurs* **18**: 384–387.

18. Manns BJ, Taub K, *et al.* (2005) The impact of education on chronic kidney disease patients. Plans to initiate dialysis with self-care dialysis: A randomized trial. *Kidney Int* **68**:1777–1783.

19. Pombo AP, Hopman WM, Meers C, McMurray M, Seriger M. (2000) The expansion of a self-care hemodialysis program due to improved outcomes. *Abstr Acad Health Serv Res Health Policy Meet* **17**.

20. Baillod RA, Comty CM, Crochelt R, Shaldon S. (1966) Experience with regular hemodialysis in the home. *EDTA Proc* **3**: 126.

21. Saran R, Bragg-Grisham JL, *et al.* (2003) Non-adherence in hemodialysis: Associations with mortality, hospitalization, and practice patterns in the DOPPS. *Kidney Int* **64**: 254–262.

22. Curtin RB, Oberley ET, *et al.* (1996) Differences between employed and non-employed dialysis patients. *Am J Kidney Dis* **27**: 533–540.

23. Shaldon S, Cantab MD. (1968) Independence in maintenance dialysis. *Lancet* 520–523.

24. Holland M, Myers G. (2007) Increasing self-care dialysis adoption. http://www.aakp.org/aakp-library/selfcare-dialysis.

25. Latham CE. (1998) Is there data to support the concept that educated, empowered patients have better outcomes? *J Am Soc Nephrol* **9**: S141–S144.

CHAPTER 7

Opting for Death Rather than Dialysis in Chronic Renal Failure

*Anthony J. Joseph**

Historical Perspectives

In its 2008 annual report, the United States Renal Data System (USRDS) noted that over 350,000 patients with end-stage renal disease (ESRD) were treated with maintenance hemodialysis (MHD) in 2006.[1] Currently, MHD is so accessible in the US that it is even offered to undocumented immigrants in several states — New York, for example. By contrast, MHD was generally unavailable for several years after its inception. When Belding H. Scribner started dialysis therapy for chronic uremia in January 1962, the University of Washington in Seattle could only afford a three-bed artificial kidney center with nurses providing nocturnal dialysis for 10–12 h twice weekly.[2] Scribner employed Kiil dialyzers and refrigerated dialysate from tanks made by Sweden Freezer, a local soft ice-cream machine manufacturer.[3] Allocating patients to this then scarce, lifesaving therapy was challenging and raised major ethical issues. Which ESRD patients should be treated? Should MHD be offered to the sickest, youngest, oldest, wealthiest, or most productive individuals? Scribner and his colleagues established two distinct boards whose mission was to select subjects who should receive MHD.[4,5] The first

*Assistant Professor of Medicine, Director, Acute Hemodialysis Unit, State University of New York at Brooklyn, Downstate Medical Center, USA.
Email: anthony.joseph@downstate.edu

panel, consisting of nephrologists, searched for stable, emotionally mature, uremic adults under the age of 45 without a long-standing history of hypertension and vascular complications. Having diabetes prevented acceptance for dialysis care. Furthermore, to be dialysis-eligible, those candidates should have been slowly deteriorating with progressive renal failure and must have demonstrated willingness to deal with the harshness of dialysis and dietary regimens. Children and young adults who could not support themselves were automatically excluded. After the first committee approval, ESRD patients meeting these strict medical criteria were referred to an anonymous board, called the Admissions and Policy Committee (APC), which included five lay members selected from varied social and economic classes, a clergyman, and a physician who was not a nephrologist. During the first 13 months of its operation, the APC evaluated 30 candidates chosen by the panel of renal physicians. Although the APC concluded that 17 were suitable to join the MHD program, only 10 were selected, while the remaining 7 died. In summary, 20 out of 30 ESRD patients screened by nephrologists and referred to the APC were not provided access to a dialysis regimen.[4,5] The critical constraint on treating all who might benefit was the cost of the new therapy. It is not surprising that the ethical stresses in Seattle provoked an article published in *Life* magazine by Shana Alexander in November 1962 describing the APC, as well a 1965 NBC documentary entitled *Who Shall Live?* These media portrayals sparked fierce criticism and generated ethical concerns over the critical selective practice.[6,7] Choosing arbitrarily who should live and who should die and sustained political activism pushed Congress to enact legislation providing almost universal Medicare entitlement to patients with ESRD requiring MHD and for kidney transplantation.[8,9] President Richard Nixon signed the legislation on the 30th of October, 1972.

By 1973, although the equipment shortage was lessening, patients with ESRD caused by diabetic nephropathy continued to be excluded from Medicare-funded MHD programs, through 1980. Excessive mortality and morbidity in diabetic dialysis patients attributed to cardiovascular, cerebrovascular, and peripheral arterial diseases encouraged such biased systems. Indeed, early studies of dialysis outcome in diabetic patients (mainly type 1 diabetes) from the US reported a two-year survival ranging from 25% to 40%.[10–12]

Until recently, in several European countries, elderly people with ESRD shared the misfortune of the Seattle pioneers and aforementioned patients with diabetic nephropathy. In 1982, G.M. Berlyne criticized the British National Health Service for its failure in providing adequate dialysis facilities for older patients: "Over 50 and uremic equals death."[13] In a survey of French nephrologists published in 1993, 90% reported refusing to dialyze individuals ≥75 years if they were not independent and lacked a supportive family.[14] Concerns have been raised about the appropriateness of biomedicalization of, and allocation of limited financial resources to, the care of elderly patients.[15]

Currently, reports from North America and industrialized European countries indicate that, ironically, patients with chronic kidney disease (CKD) or ESRD now sometimes refuse renal replacement therapy (RRT) — which comprises hemodialysis, peritoneal dialysis (PD), and kidney transplantation — and opt for death.[1] Family members and physicians may decide to withhold RRT from severely ill individuals with ESRD and acute kidney injury (AKI) on grounds of futility. In this chapter, we review the scope of the problem, the medical, ethical, and legal aspects of withholding or withdrawing dialysis, and the palliative care of uremic patients awaiting death.

Scope of the Problem

Over the past 30 years, solid epidemiologic data have illustrated the prevalence of deaths caused by or after withdrawing from dialysis (WD).[16–20] Between 1988 and 1990, WD was, in the US, the third most frequently reported primary cause of death in dialysis patients (8.4%), following cardiovascular and infectious diseases (37.1% and 12.9%, respectively).[18] In 1990, the Health Care Financing Administration introduced a new ESRD death notification form (HCFA-2746) which removed WD as a cause of death, asking whether WD occurred before death. Additionally, the possible causes of death that physicians could specify increased from 22 to 59, permitting a better understanding of ESRD mortality. Using the USRDS database, Leggat and colleagues reported that 17.8% of 116,829 deaths of ESRD patients occurring from 1990 to 1995 were preceded by WD.[20] The sharp increase in the proportion of individuals dying after WD, from 8.4% during 1988–1990 to 17.8% during 1990–1995, was attributed to the change in reporting with the new death notification form.[20]

WD has remained a major correlate of mortality among American ESRD patients. According to the 2008 USRDS report, during 2005–2006, 23.9% of 126,907 deceased patients withdrew from dialysis compared with 20.8% during 2000–2001.[1] This new upward trend is driven by better reporting due to further revision of the death notification form in 2004 and by education efforts of the American Society of Nephrology (ASN) and the Renal Physicians Association (RPA).[1,21] Two well-chronicled cases of refusal or discontinuation of MHD might also have impacted both family members' and patients' decisions. Australia's richest man, Kerry Packer, a media mogul and famous gambler, instructed his doctors not to prolong his life with dialysis when his kidney transplant failed. He died at the age of 68, in 2005.[22] Art Buchwald, Pulitzer Prize–winning columnist and author, when he was an 80-year-old diabetic, suffering from kidney failure, discontinued dialysis in February 2006 and abandoned his hospice to survive for 11 months, recounting his experience in his last book, *Too Soon to Say Goodbye*.[23]

Registries from other industrialized countries reported similar statistics. In its 11th annual report, completed in December 2008, the United Kingdom Renal Registry (UKRR) indicated that WD was the third-largest cause of death (after cardiac diseases and infections) in 2007 and accounted for 14% of deaths among all age groups.[24] It should be noted that UKRR data completeness regarding causes of death is flawed, listing less than 50% of all deaths and decreased in recent years.[24] In reporting causes of death, the Australian and New Zealand Data (ANZDATA) Registry labels as "social causes" WD deaths associated with various comorbidities, particularly malignancy and cardiovascular diseases. Among the Australian prevalent patients, in 2007, both "social causes" and cardiovascular diseases accounted for 36% of deaths. During the same year, 23% of New Zealanders on dialysis discontinued their treatment.[25] Birmele *et al.*, in a small-scale retrospective study conducted on 1436 French subjects treated with MHD and published in 2004, found that over 20% of subjects died after terminating dialysis therapy.[26] In that report, WD was the leading cause of death, followed by cardiovascular disease (18.4%).

Clinical Aspects of WD: Factors

Failure to thrive (FTT), chronic medical or serious comorbidities, female gender, sociocultural factors, and old age are associated with a higher rate of WD. In 1997, using the USRDS database, Leggat *et al.* showed that death secondary to WD occurred more frequently in women than men, in older than younger age groups, and twice as often in Caucasians as in African-Americans or Asians. Caucasian patients affected by diabetes withdrew 1.8 times as often as nondiabetic whites, while black diabetic patients discontinued their dialysis 2.3 times as often as nondiabetic Afro-Americans.[20] Individuals who suffered from chronic diseases (e.g. dementia or malignancy) were more likely to stop dialysis before death, whereas patients afflicted by acute illnesses were less likely to withdraw. Moreover, data from the 2008 USRD annual report revealed that: (a) WD increased most for patients aged 75 and older; (b) native Americans along with whites were more likely to withdraw than patients of other races; (c) FTT, a diagnosis that implied cachexia, inability to function independently, and was applied to patients with dementia, was the most common cause of withdrawal. Compared to those who died in the hospital, more patients dying at home withdrew because of FTT (36% vs. 47%, respectively). "Medical complications," however, were the most common reason given for withdrawal in those dying in the hospital (41.0% vs. 20.8%).[1]

When patients indicate that they want to terminate dialysis, it is important to ascertain their decision-making capacity. Then, it is the responsibility of renal specialists and dialysis staff members to find out why certain individuals with ESRD decide to discontinue MHD.

Identifying persons with whom they may wish to discuss their decision to stop dialysis can be invaluable to patients and the health care team. Determining which factors contributed to WD is important because, at times, nephrologists can modify dialysis prescriptions to accommodate selected patient wishes. MHD can even be initiated on a trial basis for a new patient who fears dialysis. Furthermore, for some uremic diabetic patients in whom vascular access sites have been exhausted or those with severe dialysis-associated hypotension and angina related to coronary artery disease, discussions on the potential advantages of peritoneal dialysis may induce a change of decision about WD. The prospect of a living-related kidney transplant or a simultaneous pancreas–kidney transplant can cause young diabetic patients to alter their perspective on further life. Depression, chronic pain, and disruption of quality of life are linked to WD. ESRD patients may end their desire to stop their life-sustaining treatment when specific clinical impediments to rehabilitation are removed and quality of life improves.

In ESRD patients, depression is a serious psychiatric complication linked to the false perception that ESRD and MHD must interfere with important life domains.[27] Clearly, MHD requires a considerable investment of time and significantly interrupts social, vocational, and familial tasks. Perceived intrusiveness is significantly greater in dialysis patients reporting a higher depressed mood than in other subjects. Research conducted on non-ESRD populations inferred a relationship between depression and an increased desire for death.[28] McDade-Montez *et al.*, using the Beck Depression Inventory (BDI), sought an association between a patient's level of depressive symptoms and the decision to forego MHD.[29] Patient depression correlated significantly with a decision to terminate life-sustaining dialysis. Subjects with relatively high scores on the nonsomatic subset of the BDI had a 36.4% increased risk of withdrawing from dialysis over an average period of 48 months.

In 6987 hemodialysis patients, randomly selected from dialysis centers in 12 countries, the Dialysis Outcomes and Practice Patterns Study (DOPPS II) assessed depressive symptoms using the short version of the Center for Epidemiological Studies Depression

Screening Index (CES-D).[30] A CES-D score ≥10 was indicative of depression. Higher scores implied greater depressive symptoms. Physician-diagnosed depression was noted in the medical records of 13.9% of patients. By contrast, the percentage of study participants with a CES-D score ≥10 (40%) was approximately three times higher than the prevalence of physician-diagnosed depression. DOPPS II also revealed that, compared with lower scores, a CES-D score ≥10 was associated with a 55% higher relative risk of WD. Another key finding of the analysis was how strongly comorbidities such as congestive heart failure, peripheral vascular disease, gastrointestinal bleeding, and neurological disease were associated with the rate of depressive symptoms.

Although depression is highly prevalent among hemodialysis patients, it is undertreated. Among individuals with physician-diagnosed depression and CES-D scores ≥10, 34.9% and 17.3%, respectively, had antidepressants prescribed for them.[30] An anti-depressive drug regimen may relieve depressive symptoms and improve quality of life.[31] Moderate or severe depression in older Australian patients is associated with a high degree of refusal of life-sustaining treatments, including dialysis. Management of their depression leads to increased acceptance of those life-saving therapies.[32] Evidence supports the view that individuals with ESRD contemplating WD should be referred promptly to a psychiatrist for evaluation. Furthermore, psychiatrists, particularly consultant psychiatrists, have expertise in assessing psychopathology in the presence of medical disease, determining patients' capacity to participate in medical decisions, communicating with patients, families, and staff, and negotiating complex biopsychosocial problems. Therefore, consultant psychiatrists may play a key role in helping physicians and patients deal with the ethical and legal aspects of WD discussed below.

Approximately 50% of MHD subjects complain of pain that is frequently associated with depression and consideration of WD. For example, in a cross-sectional study of 205 Canadian dialysis patients, the prevalence of depression was higher in people with moderate or severe pain compared to those with mild or no pain (34.1% vs. 18%).

Consideration of WD was significantly associated with moderate or severe chronic pain compared to no or mild pain (46% vs. 16.7%).[33]

In ESRD patients, pain may be due to musculoskeletal ailments such as osteoarthritis and renal osteodystrophy, or peripheral vascular disease, neuropathy, carpal tunnel syndrome, polycystic kidney disease, or malignancy. The character, aggravating factors, and intensity of pain should be defined. Prescribing nonnarcotic or narcotic drugs with an adjuvant from the anticonvulsant or tricyclic antidepressant group of drugs may enhance analgesia while minimizing opioid dosage and side effects. Difficult cases should be referred to a physician specializing in pain management.

Although subadequate dialysis treatment, recurrent intradialytic hypotension, excruciating cramping, pruritus, poor sleep quality, and long travel time to the dialysis unit have not been reported as direct causes of WD, they may nevertheless have a profound effect on health-related quality of life (HR-QOL). Sleep disturbance and long travel time are not frequently addressed by practicing nephrologists. Poor sleep quality is common among dialysis patients and is independently associated with several HR-QOL indices, medication use patterns, and mortality.[34] Moreover, sleep disturbance in MHD patients is closely related to depression.[35] Assessment and management of sleep quality should be an important component of care in individuals on MHD. Excessive time required to travel to dialysis treatments adds a considerable burden on hemodialysis patients. Longer travel time is significantly associated with greater mortality risk and decreased HR-QOL.[36] Traveling for more than 60 min has a 10% greater risk of WD compared with a travel time of 15 min or less.[36] Consequently, it is better to refer patients to dialysis centers located in their neighborhood unless they want to be followed by their nephrologist regardless of the practice location.

Data concerning the prevalence of WD among ESRD patients treated with PD or home hemodialysis are scanty. In a study comparing QOL, mental health factors such as anxiety and depression, and health beliefs in 77 MHD patients vs. 58 subjects on PD, Ginieri-Coccossis *et al.* found that QOL and mental health of subjects on long-term MHD were more seriously compromised than in those on

PD.[37] Fong and colleagues compared QOL and illness intrusiveness in patients treated with nocturnal home hemodialysis (NHD) (36 patients) versus PD (58 patients).[38] Similar QOL, depressive symptoms, and illness intrusiveness scores were observed among well NHD and PD patients. Although factors linked to WD have been compared in patients treated with MHD or NHD versus subjects on PD, WD was not noted in those cohorts.

Legal and Ethical Aspects of WD

Many factors in the decision to stop dialysis are intertwined. The key objective is to identify and treat them. If serious attempts have been made to treat depression, sleep disturbance, and improve HR-QOL and if the patients are mentally competent and understand the consequences of their decision, they have the legal and ethical right not to start or to discontinue dialysis. Family members or legal guardians may intervene on behalf of people who are demented or incompetent.

In the US, several prominent court decisions have consistently supported the right of patients and families to terminate life support treatment. The Karen Ann Quinlan case (referred to as the "right to die"), decided by the New Jersey Supreme Court in 1976, and the Supreme Court decision in 1990 for the Nancy Cruzan case have highlighted the principle of patient autonomy.[39,40] The Patient Self-Determination Act of 1990, written in response of the case of Cruzan, protects by federal statute the right of patients to consent to or to refuse any medical treatment, including dialysis.[41] All states sanction refusal by competent people, and most states allow surrogates to refuse treatment on behalf of incompetent patients.

Withholding and withdrawing dialysis should take place only with consent of the patient or the designated health care decision-makers. In the course of clinical care of a critically ill patient, it may become obvious that the patient is dying, and further treatment will only prolong the active dying process. At this stage, further therapeutic intervention is often described as "futile." The Council on Ethical and Judicial Affairs (CEJA) of the American Medical Association finds great difficulty in assigning an absolute definition to the term "futile care," since it is inherently a value-laden determination.[42] CEJA favors a fair process approach to determining and subsequently withholding or withdrawing treatment considered to be futile.

The principle of autonomy is not restricted to medical patients. Physicians also have the right to exercise their ethical beliefs, including the determination that a specific medical treatment such as dialysis would not benefit a patient. Hirsch and colleagues suggest that dialysis is inappropriate for patients with a poor prognosis, including those with multiple-organ system failure, metastatic and refractory malignancy, or debilitating neurologic disease.[43] Joint decision-making using outcome data and value judgments should occur between patient/proxy and physician to the greatest extent possible. Serious attempts should be made to settle differences and reach a solution within all parties' acceptable limits, with the assistance of consultants or ethics committees. CEJA recommends the transfer of care to another physician within the institution when the ethics committee endorses the patient's position. Conversely, if the ethics committee agrees with the physician's viewpoint and the patient/surrogate cannot be convinced, arrangements for transfer to another institution may be sought.[42] Physicians should not use the concept of medical futility and, unilaterally, withhold or discontinue RRT without the patients' knowledge, or over the patients' or surrogates' disagreement. If transfer is not possible because no physician and no institution can be found to follow the patient's and/or proxy's wishes, by ethics standards, futile treatment can be halted.[42] The legal ramifications of this course of action are unclear.[44]

Because WD is prevalent in the US, renal divisions and dialysis centers should be ready to deal with this stressful situation. Nephrologists should discuss advance care planning early in their relationship with patients. Studies have shown that advance care planning facilitates decision-making related to initiating and withdrawing dialysis. Over the past 20 years, the renal community has made significant progress regarding end-of-life care. Holley and colleagues reported that nephrologists surveyed in 2005 had significantly changed their practices about end-of-life care since 1990.[45] Currently, they were more likely to honor patients' wishes to

discontinue dialysis, to consult a Network Ethics Committee in difficult situations, and to have in their dialysis unit written policies on
cardiopulmonary resuscitation and dialysis withdrawal. More than
50% of those physicians indicated that they relied on "shared
decision-making in the appropriate initiation of and withdrawal from
dialysis," a clinical practice guideline developed by the RPA and the
ASN in conjunction with representatives from multiple disciplines
and organizations in the dialysis community, kidney patients and
family members, and internal medicine physicians, as well as a
bioethicist and a public policy expert.[21]

The guideline includes nine recommendations:

(1) Shared decision-making
(2) Informed consent or refusal
(3) Estimating prognosis
(4) Conflict resolution
(5) Advance directives
(6) Withholding or withdrawing dialysis
(7) Special patient groups
(8) Time-limited trials
(9) Palliative care

Palliative Care for People Refusing Dialysis and Opting for Death

After discontinuation of dialysis, most patients die within ten
days.[46,47] When there is time to plan, patients deciding to discontinue dialysis should be referred to a palliative care service. Palliative
care can be provided at home or in a nursing home or hospital.
Patients should have a "very good death," characterized as being
painless, peaceful, brief, and happening in the company of loved
ones.[47,48] A good death minimizes the distress of family and staff
members. Symptoms such as pain, nausea, vomiting, and pruritus
should be relieved. A decreased protein intake minimizes uremic
symptoms, while a restricted fluid intake can prevent fluid overload
in those with anuria. Dying of pulmonary edema is a "bad death."

Should pulmonary edema resistant to diuretics occur, a short session of ultrafiltration may be offered to restore comfort.

Refusal to start or WD is common, making it important for renal physicians to learn what encourages an ESRD patient to terminate dialysis. Depression, chronic pain, and poor HR-QOL, known associates of WD, can be treated or improved. If competent patients remain convinced of their desire to decline or discontinue dialysis after serious attempts to treat depression, relieve pain, and improve HR-QOL, the renal team should make arrangements for an easy death. After discussion regarding the consequences of refusal or WD, referral to a palliative care service optimizes the chances of a "very good death."

References

1. United States Renal Data System. (2008) USRDS 2008 annual data report. National Institutes of Health, National Institute of Diabetes and Digestive and Kidney Diseases, Bethesda, MD.
2. Murray JS, Tu WH, Albers JB, *et al*. (1962) A community dialysis center for the treatment of chronic uremia. *Trans Am Soc Artif Intern Organs* **8**: 315–319.
3. Frost TH, Jolly D, Kerr DNS. (1973) Effect of membrane grain orientation on *in vitro* performance of a Kiil dialyzer. *Kidney Int* **3**: 186–189.
4. Lindholm DD, Burnell JM, Murray JS. (1963) Experience in the treatment of chronic uremia in an outpatient community hemodialysis center. *Trans Am Soc Artif Intern Organs* **9**: 2–9.
5. Blagg CR. (2007) The early history of dialysis for chronic renal failure in the United States: a view from Seattle. *Am J Kidney Dis* **49**(3): 482–496.
6. Alexander S. (1962) They decide who lives, who dies: medical miracle puts moral burden on a small committee. *Life* **53**: 102–125.
7. Reshner N. (1969) The allocation of exotic medical lifesaving therapy. *Ethics* **79**: 173–186.
8. Rettig RA. (1976) The policy debate on patient care financing for victims of end-stage renal disease. *Law Contemp Probl* **40**(4): 196–230.
9. Rettig RA. (1991) Origins of the Medicare kidney disease entitlement: The social security amendment of 1972. In: Hanna KE (ed.), *Biomedical Politics*, pp. 176–214. National Academy Press, Washington DC.

10. Comty CM. (1971) Management and prognosis of diabetic patients treated by chronic hemodialysis. *J Am Soc Nephrol* **5**: 15.
11. Comty CM, Kjellsen D, Shapiro FL. (1976) A reassessment of the prognosis of diabetic patients treated by chronic hemodialysis. *Trans Am Soc Artif Intern Organs* **22**: 404.
12. Ghavamian M. Gutch CF, Kopp KF, Kolff WJ. (1972) The sad truth about hemodialysis in diabetic nephropathy. *JAMA* **222**: 1386–1389.
13. Berlyne GM. (1982) Over 50 and uremia equals death. The failure of the British National Health Service to provide adequate dialysis facilities. *Nephron* **31**(3): 189–190.
14. Mignon F, Michel C, Mentre F, Viron B. (1993) Worlwide demographics and future trends of the management of renal failure in the elderly. *Kidney Int Suppl* **41**: S18–S26.
15. Smith II GP. (2002) Allocating health care resources to the elderly. *Elder Law Rev* **9**: 21.
16. Neu S, Kjellstrand CM. (1986) An empirical study of withdrawal of life-supporting treatment. *N Engl J Med* **314**(1): 14–20.
17. Port FK, Wolfe RA, Hawthorne VM, Ferguson CW. (1989) Discontinuation of dialysis therapy as a cause of death. *Am J Nephrol* **9**(2): 145–149.
18. United States Renal Data System. (1993) USRDS 1993 annual data report. *Am J Kidney Dis* **22**(2).
19. Mailloux LU, Belluci AG, Napolitano B, *et al.* Death by withdrawal from dialysis: A 20-year clinical experience. *J Am Soc Nephrol* **3**: 1631–1637.
20. Leggat JE Jr, Bloembergen WE, Levine G, *et al.* (1997) Analysis of risk factors for withdrawal from dialysis before death. *J Am Soc Nephrol* **8**: 1755–1763.
21. Galla JH. (2000) Renal Physicians Association/American Society of Nephrology Working Group, Washington DC: Clinical practice guidelines on shared decision-making in the appropriate initiation of and withdrawal from dialysis. *J Am Soc Nephrol* **11**: 1340–1342.
22. Hogan J. (2005) Kerry Packer dies. *The Sydney Morning Herald*, smh.com.au, Dec 27.
23. Folkenflik D. (2007) Columnist Art Buchwald leaves us laughing. NPR.org, Jan 18.
24. Ansell D, Roderick P, Hodsman A, *et al.* (2009) UK Renal Registry 11th Annual Report (Dec 2008). Chap. 7: Survival and causes of death of UK

adult patients on renal replacement therapy in 2007: National and centre-specific analyses. *Nephron Clin Pract* **111**(1): c113–c139.

25. Australia and New Zealand Dialysis and Transplant Registry. ANZDATA 2008 annual data report (31st annual report). http://www.anzdata.org.au/v1/report_2008.html

26. Birmele B, Francois M, Pengloan J, *et al.* (2004) Death after withdrawal from dialysis: the most common of death in French dialysis population. *Nephrol Dial Transplant* **19**(3): 686–691.

27. Devins GM, Binik YM, Hutchinson TA, *et al.* The emotional impact of end-stage renal disease: Importance of patients' perceptions of intrusiveness and control. *Int J Psychiatry* **13**: 327–343.

28. Breitbart W, Rosenfeld B, Pessin H, *et al.* (2000) Depression, hopelessness, and desire for hastened death in terminally patients with cancer. *JAMA* **284**: 2907–2911.

29. McDade-Montez EA, Christensen AJ, Cvengros JA, Lawton WJ. (2006) The role of depression symptoms in dialysis withdrawal. *Health Psychol* **2**: 198–204.

30. Lopes AA, Albert JM, Young EW, *et al.* (2004) Screening for depression in hemodialysis patients: Associations with diagnosis, treatment, and outcomes in the DOPPS. *Kidney Int* **66**: 2047–2053.

31. Turk S, Atalay H, Altintepe L, *et al.* (2006) Treatment with antidepressive drugs improved quality of life in chronic hemodialysis patients. *Clin Nephrol* **65**(2): 113–118.

32. Hooper SC, Vaughan KJ, Tennant CC, Perz JM. (1996) Major depression and refusal of life-sustaining medical treatment in the elderly. *Med J Aust* **165**: 416–419.

33. Davidson SN. (2003) Pain in hemodialysis patients: prevalence, cause, severity, and management. *Am J Kidney Dis* **42**(6): 1239–1247.

34. Elder SJ, Pisoni RL, Akizawa T, *et al.* (2008) Sleep quality predicts quality of life and mortality risk in hemodialysis patients: Results from the Dialysis Outcomes and Practice Patterns Study (DOPPS). *Nephrol Dial Transplant* **23**: 998–1004.

35. Paparrigopoulos T, Theleritis C, Tzavara C, Papadaki A. (2009) Sleep disturbance in haemodialysis patients is closely related to depression. *Gen Hosp Psychiatry* **31**: 175–177.

36. Moist LM, Bragg-Gresham JL, Pisoni RL, *et al.* (2008) Travel time to dialysis as a predictor of health-related quality of life, adherence, and

mortality: The Dialysis Outcomes and Practice Patterns Study (DOPPS). *Am J Kidney Dis* **51**(4): 641–650.

37. Ginieri-Coccossis M, Theofilou P, Synodinou C, *et al.* (2008) Quality of life, mental health and health beliefs in haemodialysis and peritoneal patients: Investigating differences in early and later years of current treatment. *BMC Nephrol* **9**: 14.

38. Fong E, Bargman JM, Chan CT. (2007) Cross-sectional comparison of quality of life and illness intrusiveness in patients who are treated with nocturnal home dialysis versus peritoneal dialysis. *Clin J Am Soc Nephrol* **2**: 1195–1200.

39. Gostin LO. (1997) Deciding life and death in the courtroom: From Quinlan to Cruzan, Glucksberg, and Vacco — a brief history and analysis of constitutional protection of the "right to die." *JAMA* **278**(18): 1523–1528.

40. Crusan v Director, Missouri Department of Health, 497 U.S. 261, 110 S. Ct. 2841, 111L.ED.224 (1990).

41. Annas G. (1990) Nancy Cruzan and the right to die. *N Engl J Med* **323**: 670–673.

42. Council on Ethical and Judicial Affairs, American Medical Association. (1999) Medical futility in end-of-life care: Report of the Council on Ethical and Judicial Affairs. *JAMA* **281**(10): 937–941.

43. Hirsch DJ, West ML, Cohen AD, Jindal KK. (1994) Experience with not offering dialysis to patients with a poor prognosis. *Am J Kidney Dis* **23**(3): 463–466.

44. In the matter of Baby K, 16F3d 590 (4th Cir 1994).

45. Holley JL, Davison SN, Moss AH. (2007) Nephrologists' changing practices in reported end-of-life decision-making. *Clin J Am Soc Nephrol* **2**: 107–111.

46. Fissel RB, Bragg-Gresham JL, Lopes AA, *et al.* (2005) Factors associated with "do not resuscitate" orders and rates of withdrawal from hemodialysis in international DOPPS. *Kidney Int* **68**: 1282–1288.

47. Cohen LM, McCue J, Germain M, Kjellstrand CM. (1995) Dialysis discontinuation: A good death? *Arch Intern Med* **155**: 42–47.

48. Cohen LM, Poppel DM, Cohn GM, Reiter GS. (2001) A very good death: Measuring quality of dying in end-stage renal disease. *J Palliat Med* **4**(2): 167–172.

CHAPTER 8

Ethical Concerns in Marketing Kidneys

*Amy L. Friedman**

Background

More than half a century has passed since Joseph Murray and his team of pioneers fulfilled the promise of clinical human transplantation. Their accomplishment in successfully replacing one person's failed organ with a healthy human body part heralded a new era.[1] They had transformed the human body into a potential reservoir of spare parts for the physical repair and benefit of another individual and moved this specific realm of science fiction into reality. Though Murray had proven the concept, broad application of these medically marvelous skills did not become immediately feasible. During the subsequent years numerous other notable medical and scientific accomplishments (such as immunosuppressive regimens that result in acute rejection rates as low as 10–15 % in the first year)[2] facilitated the evolution of transplantation into our current era. Today, thanks also to the availability and financial support of dialysis, the average citizen of a developed country no longer considers renal failure a fatal prognosis. Indeed, that citizen is empowered to select a renal replacement therapy. In the United States, providers are even required to annually consider his or her suitability for transplantation, because of its identification as the most cost-effective therapy.[3] In making that choice, the average person feels entitled to unfettered

*Professor of Surgery, Director of Transplantation, SUNY Upstate Medical University, 750 East Adams Street, Syracuse, New York, 13104, USA.
Email: amy.friedman@yale.edu

access to kidney transplantation, the modality that has become the standard of care.

It is precisely the success in performing kidney transplantation for a range of persons who would never have been imagined to be reasonable candidates by those first pioneers that best illustrates the greatest irony of transplantation. We would be capable of accomplishing many more transplants than occur, but cannot do so without sufficient availability of suitable organs. Today, we routinely successfully transplant people as old as 80 years[4] or as morbidly obese as having a BMI of 45,[5] as well as those with diabetes and those infected with the human immunodeficiency virus.[6] Even active but slow-growing malignancy may not always preclude *de novo* renal transplantation.[7] In fact, the only true contraindication is a medical or psychosocial condition judged to be likely to limit the candidate's longevity to less than 2–3 years or to make followup care too uncontrolled to facilitate patient safety, as in the case of noncompliance.

So, the modern tragedy has become the increasingly disproportionate number of suitable kidney transplant candidates and the stagnant, meager supply of kidneys to offer them. For increasing numbers of patients, legitimate transplantation is like a promised land that can be seen but never personally experienced. Though deemed suitable candidates, these patients will die without receiving a transplant.

Ethics of the Organ Transplant Center in an Organ Shortage

American transplant centers have been dually designated to perform the transplant candidate selection process and to be responsible for directly delivering to the patients the bad news about this dismal situation. Though nephrologists and dialysis teams effectively serve as the gatekeepers to the world of transplantation for the majority of ESRD patients, regulatory agencies — e.g. Centers for Medicare and Medicaid Services (CMS) and the Organ Procurement and Transplant Network (OPTN) — have specifically stipulated multiple elements of the transplant patient education process, and have imposed explicit related requirements, placing the transplant team squarely in charge of delivering these ominous data.[8,9] For example, transplant teams are required to notify patients in writing within ten business days of formal evaluation whether or not they have been placed on the waiting list, together with the center's rationale for doing so. While a nephrologist may completely avoid confronting the patient with his or her projected mortality, the transplant team cannot do so. Among the outcome data that patients must be given are the rates of transplantation and mortality for those placed on the waiting list. These data are now publicly available for each US transplant center, and patients are encouraged to review them regularly.[10] Transplant center personnel have thus been left "holding the bag" and are expected to explain society's failure to resolve the organ shortage to the very patients seeking their help.

Little has been written about the modern day burden which transplant team members assume in playing this role. By extension from the early days of dialysis, when participants in the "who shall live and who shall die" type committees suffered lasting personal trauma from their role in the allocation of scarce dialysis slots,[11] one might expect to encounter significant adverse consequences for the transplant teams themselves. Whether the performance of stressful tasks (patient selection and education) ultimately translates into suboptimal human ethical behaviors by transplant providers is unknown. Certainly, however, these very human personnel can be expected to be subject to all of the frailties and imperfections of the human condition. One should not expect them to remain unaffected.

Consider the example of transplant surgeons who demonstrate intrinsic bias against selecting patients afflicted with specific disease states despite familiarity with data supportive of unaffected rates of associated adverse outcomes. Thus, HIV is generally viewed as a contraindication, even though these patients have similar posttransplant survival to HCV-infected patients who are considered appropriate candidates.[12] One must wonder about the relative impacts of the organ shortage, the individual provider's expertise in management of specific disease states and even the extent and/or

nature of that provider's personal interaction with the hopeful transplant candidate as such life or death decisions are made.

Indeed, the process used by transplant centers to select patients
and select organs remains, to a great degree, subjective. Despite the
regulatory requirement to establish, follow and document a
transplant-specific patient selection policy (see above), many relevant factors contribute to the center's final determination, which is
essentially a judgment call. For this reason, the same patient may be
declined at one center and accepted at another.

Virtually unexplored in a substantive way is the issue of the
center's overlapping roles and the conflicts of interest naturally
engendered (Fig. 1). On one hand, the transplant team addresses
patient-centric issues. Thus, the team considers how to best directly
provide care for the patient together with how to advocate for the
patient within a complex system and a serious organ shortage. On
the other hand, the center-centric considerations bearing on transplant decisions include supplementation of the center's wait list
volume, growth of the number of actual transplants performed, cost

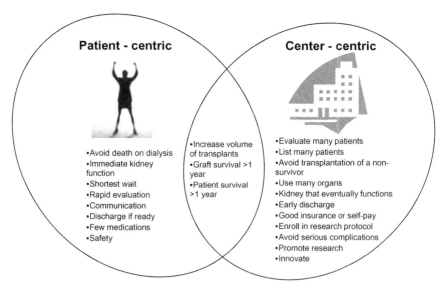

Fig. 1.   The transplant center's overlapping roles.

containment (e.g. ensuring a competitive length of stay or avoiding complex patients requiring expensive therapies), financial solvency (e.g. soliciting access to wealthy, self-paying patients; or promoting research protocols that generate fees for investigators and facilities) and meeting regulatory requirements (e.g. outcomes such as patient and graft survival).[13]

From the team's perspective, those candidates not likely to survive the projected wait time until transplantation may include relatively sick, fragile patients whose medical condition also makes them higher-risk and therefore increases the likelihood of poor outcomes after transplantation. Informally, such patients may not receive a team's wholehearted advocacy efforts. In contrast, a somatically robust patient with a very high level of circulating antibodies (preformed antibodies increase the difficulty of finding a compatible donor) might be enrolled in protocols requiring expensive products (e.g. plasmapheresis, intravenous immune globulin and/or rituxamab)[14] and meeting a center's research objectives. It is not difficult to surmise that such incentives might lead to greater team promotion of an individual's options for transplantation. All of these factors may remain unappreciated by even the savviest patient. Complete transparency, even within the team itself, may not be equally embraced at all transplant centers.

In truth, today there are numerous, complex and sometimes competing strategies for enhancing an individual's access to an organ for transplantation (Fig. 2). Although transplant teams are likely aware of the existence of all of these strategies, there may be varied enthusiasm for their pursuit, depending on the relative impact of the factors elaborated above. As in all of healthcare, the provider's obligation to fully inform a patient about all available treatment options is another incompletely explored ethical arena. If, for example, a particular strategy not developed at a specific transplant center is available at a direct competitor, or even at a geographically remote center, should the patient be offered access to it? How should the patient with compromised healthcare literacy be approached? When such a patient is unable or unwilling to become seriously engaged in the decision-making process (e.g. the patient who says, "I trust that

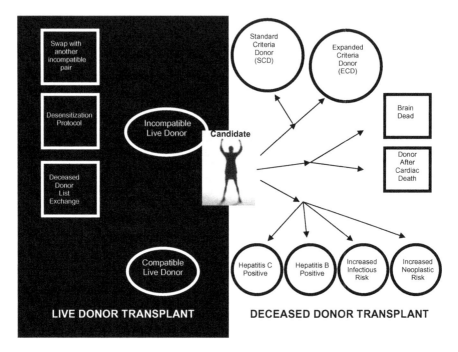

Fig. 2.   Options for the kidney transplant candidate to consider in 2009.

God will help you make the right choices"), should the same range of options be presented? Are they?

In the United States, frank assessment of the impact costs and reimbursement (or lack thereof) and how they contribute to management decisions is sobering. For the center, the indigent patient lacking any type of insurance creates difficult dilemmas. Even if the costs for (a) the initial hospitalization, (b) procurement of the organ from either a living donor or the wait list (organ acquisition cost) and (c) the initial outpatient visits can be funded, the posttransplant medication regimen will likely be incapacitating, reaching approximately US$15,000 per year.[15] Even those patients covered by Medicare must find a means of paying for 20% of immunosuppressants (Medicare covers 80% of the antirejection medications for three years) and all the standard medications (the average posttransplant patient takes 10 unique medications).[16] Consensus on whether or not a center should perform such a transplant despite knowledge that the patient's posttransplant medication coverage is insufficient has not been achieved. Those centers for whom transplant volume is the driving force, and who do not routinely continue to provide care beyond the early posttransplant period, may consider such a transplant appropriate. But other centers, who subscribe to a lifelong patient–provider contract model for providing care to their transplant recipient, may not. Concern about thrusting the ESRD patient into an unsolvable predicament, with the possible outcomes of graft loss and preclusion of a subsequent transplant (the first transplant may result in high levels of circulating antibodies), may inhibit the center's approval of the patient's candidacy. One perspective is not necessarily more ethical than another. The issues are incredibly complex. In the clearest validation of the grave, chaotic state of cost and reimbursement issues within the American renal transplant environment in 2009, UNOS and the American Society of Transplantation have just disseminated results (still unpublished) of an Internet survey of 99% of American kidney transplant centers. Their key findings were that patient inability to afford immunosuppressive medications within the current environment is common and catastrophic. More than 65% of transplant centers reported patient deaths or the failure of transplant kidneys due to cost-related medication nonadherence.

Yet another, linked ethical dilemma for the transplant center pertains to the right of a wait list candidate to be actively listed at multiple centers within the United States. In fact, all kidney transplant centers are specifically required to inform their patients of this opportunity, provide them with relevant written materials and fully document having done so.[17] The advantages of multiple listing include the individual's opportunity to seek the shortest predicted wait time for a kidney, as well as selecting a transplant center by other factors (e.g. a famous transplant surgeon or a specific research protocol). Clearly, advocating that a transplant candidate consider placement on a different transplant center's list is rarely consistent with the referring transplant team's business objectives. Among candidates, levels of perceptiveness about the benefits and feasibility of multiple listing are likely influenced by factors including their personality, intelligence, healthcare literacy, financial means, etc. It is apparent that not all patient cohorts will benefit to an equivalent extent from this practice. Similarly, multiple listing is not a strategy that most transplant centers are likely to energetically espouse, even though it may be in the patient's best interest.

Thus, it is apparent that transplant centers vary widely in their approaches to those seeking to undergo kidney transplantation for reasons that may be principally self-serving and practical. Denial of such diversity among centers would be disingenuous and fundamentally unfair to the transplant candidate. Yet, in practice, interactions between the candidate and the transplant center are generally infrequent and brief and provide minimal opportunities for individualized strategic planning. Ideally, it is most appropriate to conduct an initial, forthright discussion with the ESRD patient, to determine the patient's degree of desperation and tolerance for the unknown and unpredictable. Based on this encounter, a patient-specific management plan should be developed.

Ethics of the Transplant Candidate in an Organ Shortage

Facing these brutal realities, the patient may be confused and overwhelmed and develop a sense of hopelessness, particularly if he or she had embarked on the transplant evaluation process unprepared and/or with unrealistic expectations. How the patient reacts to this information and responds to the required medical testing and data collection typically required to reach a "transplant or don't transplant" determination is critically important. Indecision and inaction translate directly into delay and are therefore highly counterproductive.[18] For the transplant candidate, delay is the equivalent of increased mortality risk. For this reason, the ideal patient has been empowered to be assertive. Unfortunately, effective self-advocacy is difficult to establish.[19] Naivete about the dysfunctional state of the healthcare system, though comprehensible, seriously jeopardizes transplant candidacy. For example, candidates often assume that outstanding issues are being effectively handled by the team. In truth, the complexity of sharing medical data in the absence of a uniform medical record, combined with the involvement of multiple providers, is often underappreciated. Some patients seem to expect that every physician somehow becomes magically informed and collaborates in medication changes or altered therapeutic plans made by other participating providers.[20] And, in the case of such critical questions as whether or not to proceed with cardiac catheterization in a diabetic predialysis patient, deferral by a cardiologist (due to concern that the need for renal replacement therapy may be precipitated) effectively halts transplant progress.[21] Months may pass before the legitimate problem is recognized, leading to postponement of all transplant-related action, even if a suitable living donor is available.[22] Other circumstances, such as the need to definitely exclude and/or treat malignancy or opportunistic infection in a lung nodule, may require extensive collaboration between health providers — the type of care coordination that has today become increasingly challenging with the progressive reduction of practitioners' uncommitted time.

Even when an appropriate, proactive patient gains approval by a transplant center, involvement of the patient's payer often introduces further delay. Take the example of the patient who never missed or abbreviated a hemodialysis session, was compulsive about taking every dose of medication exactly as prescribed, worked at a full-time job and trustingly confided the regular use of marijuana (to combat nausea) to the transplant team. After complete evaluation the transplant social worker and team concluded that isolated use of marijuana, though an admittedly illegal method of countering stress, did not preclude transplantation for the otherwise excellent candidate. Yet, preapproval of a live donor transplant was declined by the insurance company's medical director, who insisted on documentation of a one-month abstinence period, together with multiple negative toxicology tests. In this case, the patient was penalized for honesty. He was left dependent on the transplant center's ability to successfully reverse the payer's denial. In this real case, this author did successfully advocate for the patient, by supporting the transplant center's decision with the best published evidence.[23] However, the advocacy process required nearly two weeks to complete, and forced rescheduling of a live donor transplant. Ironically, the delay increased expense, adding bureaucracy that would have been completely avoided had the patient simply lied about the use of marijuana. Little wonder that patients seeking transplantation are not always honest with the teams evaluating their candidacy.

Once transplantation is determined to be appropriate, the candidate still has other key decisions to make, all of which have unique associated ethical challenges (Table 1). The most powerful determinants of most answers are the strength of the person's ego and self-worth and the intensity of his or her desperation to have a transplant, both of which remain unstudied. To a great extent, the transplant team is responsible for educating the patient and developing informed consent about these alternatives. Yet, ultimately, the team's role is to provide valuable guidance without unilaterally making these choices. For example, while many patients who are themselves parents will decline kidneys offered by their offspring, there are occasional patients who are comfortable about accepting

Table 1.   Ethical Considerations for the Transplant Candidate

- Is there a suitable volunteer live donor?
- Will the candidate accept the live donor's offer?
- What is the chance of surviving the wait for a deceased donor's kidney within the legitimate system?
- Should a marginal organ be accepted in order to survive the wait for a kidney within the legitimate system?
- Should a high risk organ be accepted in order to survive the wait for a kidney within the legitimate system?
- Should a live donor's kidney be solicited in the US?
- Should a live donor's kidney be secretly purchased in the US?
- Should a kidney be purchased outside of the US?
- Where should the kidney be purchased?
- Who will take care of the candidate upon return to the US?
- How will the medications be paid for?

organs donated by their grandchildren. Such sensitive decisions that fall within conventional medical guidelines are beyond the jurisdiction of anyone but the donor, the recipient and their respective consciences.

The Black Market in Kidneys Circa 2009

The existence of a black market in which money is exchanged for an organ from a live donor is no longer questioned. Through combined efforts of lay journalists and medical detectives, consensus has been reached about the general description of this market.[24] In the United States, this activity is specifically defined as illegal by the National Organ Transplant Act of 1984, in Section 274e, entitled "Prohibition of Organ Purchases."[25] No such illegal transplants have been identified in any of the major countries in which transplantation is widely available. The only location in which donor compensation is legally permissible in 2009 is Iran.[26] However, payment for organs has been well documented in India, Pakistan, China, the Philippines and elsewhere. Though it is difficult to characterize completely because of the covert nature of these transplants, most agree that the majority involve indigent donors and relatively wealthy patients from developed countries in which legitimate transplantation is not immediately available (see discussions above). Third party brokers siphon off a substantial portion of payments. The unavoidable conclusion is that the organ shortage is driving the black market.

Derived mostly from reports of outcomes collected retrospectively and, to some degree, surreptitiously, the portrait emerging for care (e.g. quality and safety) provided in this market is highly disturbing. Donation has not always been voluntary, informed consent has been less than complete, outdated surgical techniques have been applied (i.e. donor nephrectomy through a conventional, open flank incision instead of a minimally invasive approach), and transparency about short and long term outcomes has been notably absent.[27] As might be expected, the healthcare professionals applying covert "practices" have violated the most basic principles of ethical medical care for those live kidney donors involved. Without question, these transplant team members have violated society's trust in healthcare providers, and should be considered criminals.

Expansion of this black market has generated important ethical quandaries for legitimate transplant centers. In 2009 the ability to practice a "don't ask, don't tell" type of policy about kidneys purchased illegally is no longer feasible. Virtually every legitimate North American transplant center has managed patients it suspected of having "acquired" kidneys on the black market. Indian, Canadian and American[28] teams have documented that patients returning with newly transplanted, purchased kidneys must be cared for without the benefit of related surgical record information about the evaluation or infectious disease profile of the donor.[29] These recipients have been found to bear significantly increased risks of life threatening infections when compared to contemporaneous local transplants, and have inferior graft and patient survival rates. Indeed, the return of these patients who feel entitled to modern transplant care essentially places the transplant team in the middle of a complicated postoperative course with serious handicaps. After much debate in the transplant community on the question of whether participation of legitimate teams in these patients' care serves to promote the black market, most have concluded that denial of high quality care would unfairly punish these patients. After all, who can really blame or penalize a patient for seeking an organ that the system itself was unable to provide, when the transplant provides life and no transplant leads to death? But the patient's prospective assumption that such specialized care will always be available is certainly disturbing, and may invoke a variety of emotional responses from those who ultimately provide it.

Even more problematic is the challenge of helping these returning patients reintegrate into the healthcare system upon their return. In America, the system exposes them to extraordinary medication costs (see above). Few of these transplant travelers are prepared to learn that Medicare does not cover the immunosuppressive medications for transplants performed at non-Medicare-approved centers.[8] Such information certainly is not shared in advance of the transplant by the black market center, and cannot be provided by a legitimate center, unless the patient is honest in advance about his or her plans for transplant tourism. In practice, such honesty is rarely encountered and would potentially introduce issues that remain essentially unexplored from many prospective sources, including prosecutors, payers and even malpractice attorneys. If such a discussion were to take place between a patient and an American physician, one might indeed wonder about the prudence of undertaking accurate documentation of its occurrence.

In practice, it seems that many of the citizens of developed countries who do seek and find organs on the black market have made substantial life choices to amass sufficient funds for this undertaking. The majority do not seem to be sufficiently wealthy that the costs of maintenance medications are truly neglible. In other words, they do become financially caught in difficult circumstances that they had not anticipated. One should not be surprised that unscrupulous schemers, even in the United States, find ways to further victimize these desperate patients. In one recent case a Syracuse, New York native who collected as much as US$70,000 for Internet-arranged black market transplants abroad never delivered them, leading to death for the patients and financial ruin for the families left behind.[30]

In response to the burgeoning black market, the World Health Organization has recently increased attempts to focus the spotlight of international attention on this issue. Through rapid identification of current black market activities and public censure, successful efforts to close down illegal donation "rings" in several areas have indeed been made. Unfortunately, as often occurs with any type of criminal activity, new activities rapidly develop in alternate locations. An associated effort to formally denounce these practices and establish consensus was convened by the Transplantation Society and the International Society of Nephrology, in 2008. The document produced at this summit, called The Declaration of Istanbul on Organ Trafficking and Transplant Tourism, has much validity.[31] No legitimate authority or expert argues that the black market can be tolerated.

The Regulated Market in Kidneys Circa 2012

The strong, intrinsic human will to live is not eliminated by development of end stage renal disease for most patients whose natural response is investment of their own personal life force in the struggle to prolong survival. Relentless growth in this pool of desperate candidates, and the common awareness of how much can be achieved through kidney transplantation (outstanding quality and quantity of life), are the true genesis of the illegal kidney market. When both the providers who appropriately make referrals for transplantation, and their patients who make superhuman efforts to comply with all advice and prescribed medications, have played by all of society's rules, yet confront insurmountable obstacles to transplantation, the system has failed. Without the organ — a viable replacement human kidney — transplantation cannot occur. And today's transplant teams are increasingly unable to deliver this life-saving therapy to a substantial proportion of the candidates they evaluate. Unless substantial progress toward resolving the shortage of legitimate organs is made, efforts to close down the black market are unlikely to succeed.

Extrapolation from historical successes in closure of other black markets, such as the manufacture and distribution of alcohol during the era of Prohibition, leads logically to the consideration of legitimizing payment for live kidney donors. To close the black market in kidneys, why not effectively eliminate the shortage driving it? If donor compensation and protection can be accomplished within the system and lead to more organ donations, why would the donors and/or their recipients seek to bypass it? Ideally, one would hope that the introduction of transparency into this transaction would improve safety for both donors and recipients and the availability of organs. Facilitation of more transplants, as well as preservation of the rights and dignity of all parties, are the key objectives. To accomplish this, the design and structure of a mechanism must follow fundamental guidelines to ensure equity, quality and ethical behavior.

Explicit prohibition of organ purchases by NOTA has not applied to the open exchange of tangibly valuable consideration for the use or transfer (permanent or temporary) of all or part of the human body in medical therapies other than transplants. Once a shocking concept, remuneration is now firmly established in other modern medical fields in the United States. Thus, compensation for blood, tissue, sperm, eggs, and use of the uterus for surrogate pregnancy, is completely legal.[32] Although provocative legal and ethical issues are still raised in relation to aspects of these payments, the basic principle that compensation for these human products is acceptable is solidly upheld within the public domain.

Still, some individuals may be only able to justify their tolerance for these exchanges by considering the direct clinical benefit delivered to another person, in effect counterbalancing the distasteful aspects of the purchase with immediacy of the accomplished good. However, when the connection between payment and improvement of the human condition is less direct, as in purchase of human products for research purposes, fewer people remain comfortable, even though the principles remain unchanged. Here too, however, the precedent for legal and ethical acceptance has been well established. As an ultimate example, in June 2009 the Empire State Stem Cell Board of New York state approved payment of state taxpayer-backed funds in compensation for women donating oocytes for research purposes.[33]

Are there any substantive differences between these other examples of acceptable payment for a human body part or product from the reproductive and/or research fields and the donation of an entire human kidney that preclude consideration of this potentially fruitful solution to the shortage of transplant organs? Listed in Table 2 are some apparent relevant distinctions. None is sufficient to justify perpetual denial of efforts to explore this option, when so many lives are at stake. In fact, there is an increasingly loud groundswell of support for pilot trials of the most palatable forms of compensation for live kidney donors, in 2009. Advocates for legalizing payment, or at least for legalizing trials of the efficacy of doing so, now include many highly respected transplant surgeons, the 1992 Nobel laureate in economics, Gary S. Becker, and the American Society of Transplant Surgeons, the American Medical

Table 2. Similarities and Distinctions Between Payment for Human Organs Used for Transplantation and Other Uses

	Risk of Procurement or Use	Potential for Replacement in Donor	Legality
Hair	−	+++	+
Blood	−	+++	+
Sperm	−	+++	+
Egg	+	−	+
Uterus (rental)	+++	−	+
Kidney	++	+	−

Association[34] and the American Association of Kidney Patients, among others.

As in any financial undertaking, concern about coercion and exploitation of specific individuals is relevant. Fortunately, robust processes specifically created to protect the rights of the volunteer living donor are well established and will serve well to guarantee that appropriate informed consent from the compensated donor is also obtained within a context of free thought and complete confidentiality. The key elements of this protective approach to the donor include (1) live donor advocacy without conflict of interest; (2) specific, independent consent processes for evaluation and donation; (3) required followup by the transplant center for a minimum of two years; and (4) required disclosure of outcome data for donors and recipients.

Within a context of full informed consent, there is no unique or valid rationale for preventing the willing participant from financial gain through his or her donation. The precedent for financial enticement in exchange for use of the human body, and the acceptance of associated risks and potential bodily harm, are ingrained in a society whose military ranks are composed of "volunteer" soldiers. Many of these recruits have accepted tuition, advanced education and other forms of compensation in exchange for the service that is gratefully accepted by their country.

Furthermore, exclusion of a donor's compensation would isolate that individual as the only party not deriving tangible benefit from his or her action. How can such a hero freely choosing to save a life at the risk of his or her own be prevented from joining all of the other parties who prosper from his or her donation, including the recipient (prolonged survival), surgeon and anesthesiologist (procedure-based fees), hospital (facility fee and reputation) and transplant administrator (transplant volume equals job validation)?

The specific form and amount of compensation appropriate to exchange for a human kidney remain controversial but should not become the focal point of debate. As shown in Table 3, most agree that the most appropriate benefit is lifelong health insurance that might, as an example, be provided through Medicare. While a variety of other specific rewards have been proposed, careful analysis of the value gained by removing the maintenance costs of the recipient's dialysis from the healthcare system suggests that a total "compensation package" worth US$95,000 would be cost-neutral and, therefore, sustainable.[35]

Transparency is the most important principle that will protect the interests of all parties. It can only be achieved through involvement of the least biased party — the government. Thus, formal housing of the organization responsible for the planning, management and ongoing evaluation of a live donor market must fall within governmental jurisdiction. In the United States, the most appropriate mechanism would be linkage of this program to the Organ

Table 3. Acceptability of Potential Incentives in Exchange for a Kidney

Acceptability	
↑	Extra Points on the Wait List (currently effective)
	Medal of Recognition
	Term Life Insurance
	Health Insurance
	Tuition Benefit
	Monetary Payment

Procurement and Transplantation Network (OPTN), which already oversees other transplant and donor-related activities. As in these other areas, data collection and analysis must be integrally incorporated into the program from the outset.

Exclusion of third parties seeking profit from the program is another requisite. To achieve this objective, uniform compensation, without the opportunity for negotiation or bias, is required, together with prohibition of supplemental "valuable exchange." The compensation must be transferred indirectly, on behalf of the donor and recipient. The ability to negotiate or alter a standard compensation must be strictly prohibited, in order to ensure that all donors and all recipients involved (even the indigent patients) are provided with equal opportunity to participate in these transplants.

Oversight, design and, as needed, revision of the entire program, amount of compensation and outcomes for all parties must be accomplished in a manner that is protected from political influence and involves input from all relevant stakeholders. To achieve this, the panel, or board, must have a multidisciplinary composition.

While some suggest that overt compensation would demean the donor and imperil human dignity,[36] current care offered to the kidney donor within the system is far from ideal and therefore neither protective nor respectful. At best, the conventional approach to these heroes is disingenuous. For example, it is widely agreed that live kidney donors should have routine checks of their blood pressure and renal function for the rest of their single-kidneyed lives. Nevertheless, knowledge that a donor does not have healthcare insurance to cover such care beyond the postoperative recovery period (during which the recipient's insurance does apply) does not preclude extirpation of the kidney.[37] Ironically, the initial access to care under the currently available systems may be more secure for the living person who donates in Iran than in the United States.

Conclusions

Transplantation may be simultaneously the most visible, scientifically remarkable, successful and yet unattainable therapy sought by the general public in the early years of the third millennium of human history. Continued focus on the glorious achievement of salvaging a small number of lives for those fortunate citizens who benefit from a system failing to serve many other average people is the sad masking of reality. Society loses in a myriad of ways, including the outright financial drains from high costs of supporting dialysis and the lost potential tax revenues from transplant recipients who might have rejoined the workforce. Such losses also constitute the spectrum of missing contributions from those people who might have been rescued through the return of good kidney function. In lieu of blaming those whose desire to live drives them to seek organs on the illicit and dangerous black market, we would be better served by concentrating on improving the safety and regulation of live donor transplantation by eclipsing their need to find kidneys that cannot be legitimately provided. The time for acknowledgment of the donor's gift of life, through appropriate and highly regulated compensation, delivered within a transparent, public, regulated market, has come. It is only through such an initiative that the true potential of renal transplantation will be fulfilled.

References

1. Murray JE. (1992) Human organ transplantation: Background and consequences. *Science* **256**: 1411–1416.
2. Humar A, Gillingham K, Kandaswamy R, *et al.* (2007) Steroid avoidance regimens: A comparison of outcomes with maintenance steroids versus continued steroid avoidance in recipients having an acute rejection episode. *Am J Transplant* **7**(8): 1948–1953.
3. http://www.cms.hhs.gov/SurveyCertificationGenInfo/downloads/SCletter08-31.pdf Accessed on 5 July 2009.
4. Macrae J, Friedman AL, Friedman EA, *et al.* (2005) Live and deceased donor kidney transplantation in patients aged 75 years and older in the United States. *Intern Urol Nephrol* **37**(3): 641–648.
5. Massarweh NN, Clayton JL, Mangum CA, *et al.* (2005) High body mass index and short- and long-term renal allograft survival in adults. *Transplantation* **80**(10): 1430–1434.

6. Locke JE, Montgomery RA, Warren DS, *et al.* (2009) Renal transplant in HIV-positive patients: Long-term outcomes and risk factors for graft loss. *Arch Surg* **144**(1): 83–86.

7. Secin FP, Carver B, Kattan MW, *et al.* (2004) Current recommendations for delaying renal transplantation after localized prostate cancer treatment: Are they still appropriate? *Transplantation* **78**: 710–712.

8. Medicare Program; hospital conditions of participation: Requirements for approval and reapproval of transplant centers to perform organ transplants. (2007) *Fed Reg* **72**(61): 15,198–16,280.

9. http://www.unos.org/policiesandBylaws2/bylaws/UNOSByLaws/pdfs/bylaw_122.pdf, accessed on 3 July 2009.

10. http://www.ustransplant.org, accessed on 3 July 2009.

11. Blagg CR. (1998) Development of ethical concepts in dialysis: Seattle in the 1960s. *Nephrology* **4**: 235–238.

12. Halpern SD, Asch DA, Shaked A, *et al.* (2005) Determinants of transplant surgeons' willingness to provide organs to patients infected with HBV, HCV or HIV. *Am J Transplant* **5**(6): 1319–1325.

13. Englesbe MJ, Ads Y, Cohn JA, *et al.* (2008) The effects of donor and recipient practices on transplant center finances. *Am J Tranpslant* **8**(3): 586–592.

14. Tanriover B, Wright SE, Foster SV, *et al.* (2008) High-dose intravenous immunoglobulin and rituximab treatment for antibody-mediated rejection after kidney transplantation: A cost analysis. *Transplant Proc* **40**(10): 3393–3396.

15. Chisholm MA, Marshall J, Smith KE, *et al.* (2008) Medicare-approved drug discount cards and renal transplant patients: How much can these cards reduce prescription costs? *Clin Transplant* **19**(3): 357–363.

16. Page TF, Woodward RS. (2008) Cost of lifetime immunosuppression coverage for kidney transplant recipients. *Health Care Fin Rev* **30**(2): 95–104.

17. http://www.unos.org/PoliciesandBylaws2/policies/pdfs/policy_4.pdf, accessed on 4 July 2009.

18. Axelrod DA, Guidinger MK, Finlayson S, *et al.* (2008) Rates of solid-organ wait-listing, transplantation, and survival among residents of rural and urban areas. *JAMA* **299**(2): 202–207.

19. Hays R, Waterman AD. (2008) Improving preemptive transplant education to increase living donation rates: Reaching patients earlier in their disease adjustment process. *Prog Transplant* **18**(4): 251–256.
20. Merkin SS, Cavanaugh K, Longenecker JC, *et al.* (2007) Agreement of self-reported comorbid conditions with medical and physician reports varied by disease among end-stage renal disease patients. *J Clin Epidemiol* **60**(6): 634–642.
21. Ramanathan V, Goral S, Tanriover B, *et al.* (2005) Screening asymptomatic diabetic patients for coronary artery disease prior to renal transplantation. *Transplantation* **79**: 1453–1458.
22. Grubbs V, Gregorich SE, Perez-Stable EJ, *et al.* (2009) Health literacy and access to kidney transplantation. *Clin J Am Soc Nephrol* **4**(1): 16–17.
23. Coffman KL. (2008) The debate about marijuana usage in transplant candidates: Recent medical evidence on marijuana health effects. *Curr Opin Organ Transplant* **13**: 189–195.
24. http://www.nytimes.com/2004/05/23/world/organ-trade-global-black-market-tracking-sale-kidney-path-poverty-hope.html, accessed on 3 July 2009.
25. http://www.unos.org/SharedContentDocuments/NOTA_as_amended_Jan_2008.pdf, accessed on 3 July 2009.
26. Friedman AL. (2008) Do we treat live donors as patients or commoditites? *Transplantation* **86**(7): 899–900.
27. http://seattletimes.nwsource.com/html/nationworld/2004153078_kidneys30.html, accessed on 3 July 2009.
28. Gill J, MAdhira BR, Gjertson D, *et al.* (2008) Transplant tourism in the United States: A single-center experience. *Clin J Am Soc Nephrol* **3**(6): 1820–1828.
29. Inston NG, Gill D, Al-Hakim A, *et al.* (2005) Living paid organ transplantation results in unacceptably high recipient morbidity and mortality. *Transplant Proc* **37**(2): 560–562.
30. http://blog.syracuse.com/east/2009/05/organ_transplant_investigation.html, accessed on 3 July 2009.
31. Participants in the International Summit on Transplant Tourism and Organ Trafficking. The Declaration of Istanbul on Organ Trafficking and Transplant Tourism. (2008) *Transplantation* **86**(8): 1013–1018.

32. Friedman AL. (2006) Payment for living organ donation should be legalized. *BMJ* **333**(7571): 746–748.
33. http://www.the-scientist.com/blog/display/55766, accessed on 3 July 2009.
34. http://www.msnbc.msn.com/id/25356966/print/1/displaymode/1098, accessed on 3 July 2009.
35. Matas AJ. (2008) Design of a regulated system of compensation for living kidney donors. *Clin Transplant* **22**: 378–384.
36. Budiani-Saberi DA, Delmonico FL. (2008) Organ trafficking and transplant tourism: A commentary on the global realities. *Am J Transplant* **8**(5): 925–929.
37. Wainright JL, Davis CL. (2008) Short-term complications in recent living kidney donors. *Am J Transplant* **8**(S2): 282.

PART 2

PROJECTED THERAPY CIRCA 2012

CHAPTER 9

The Wearable Artificial Kidney: A New Paradigm in the Treatment of ESRD

*Victor Gura**

For the last six decades, dialysis has changed kidney failure from a death sentence to a treatable condition. Yet, as more than 1, 2 million patients sustain life by subjecting themselves to different renal replacement treatments, the outcomes of end stage renal disease (ESRD) treatment remain unacceptably poor, in terms of both mortality[1] and the miserable quality of life of these patients.[2–4] Furthermore, the mortality of ESRD patients on renal replacement therapy (RRT) is similar to that for metastatic carcinomata of the breast or colon. Even though thanks to the development of RRTs the nephrology community succeeded in keeping all these patients alive for quite some time, we have plenty to do to improve the plight of these unfortunate patients in terms of both life span and life quality. Not to be ignored is that RRTs are expensive and the ever-increasing costs of and demand for medical care for ESRD make RRT one of the major cost centers of the healthcare budget of most countries.

To make things worse, there is a meteoric increase in the incidence and prevalence of ESRD in the industrialized world[1] while in Third World countries, as improvements are achieved in nutrition and standards of life, a new pandemic of ESRD is emerging, with little to offer in sight in terms of availability and affordability of RRTs.

*Attending Physician, Cedars Sinai Medical Center Associate Clinical Professor, The David Geffen School of Medicine, University of California, Los Angeles, USA.

Also, inasmuch as there is less money available to treat patients better and more of them, the number of human assets available for meeting those needs, such as adequately trained technicians and nurses, is continuously shrinking.

Therefore, from both a humanitarian and an economic point of view, the need emerges to rethink how we deliver RRTs and whether we can achieve better and more care while utilizing fewer labor resources and spending less money.

The current standard scheme of RRT is mostly implemented in the form of hemodialysis, twice or thrice weekly for 3–4 h, thus delivering a total time of blood purification therapy of approximately 9–12 h a week. Somehow, opposed to common sense, we have been convinced for decades that blood filtration for 9–12 h a week with commonly used dialysis machines will provide the same outcome delivered by two native kidneys filtering blood for 168 h a week.

Rising evidence indicates that when dialysis time is significantly increased and fluid removal is done in smaller but more frequent amounts, treatment outcomes in ESRD seem to improve. Daily administration of hemodialysis seems to be associated with numerous improvements in quality of life and potentially increased longevity of ESRD patients.[5–10] Furthermore, the sharp shifts in the electrolyte composition of plasma, interstitial and intracellular fluid compatments, as well as the rapid removal of large amounts of fluid in a very short period of time, seem to play a significant role in the cardiovascular morbidity and mortality of ESRD patients.[11,12] Physiological removal of excess fluid by native kidneys typically averages 40–70 ml/h. In comparison, the removal of 2–4 l of fluid in 3–4 h is highly "unphysiological."[13] Moreover, fast elimination of large volumes of body fluids in such a short period of time is conducive to increased cardiovascular mortality.[14] Since most of the excess fluid accumulated by ESRD patients is stored in the interstitial and intracellular compartments, the hasty contraction of the intravascular space without allowing for physiological "refilling" from the interstitial space results in hypotensive episodes and hemodynamic instability, with deleterious effects on cardiovascular health.[15] Moreover, every practicing nephrologist knows only too well how sick our patients feel after abrupt and fast removal of large amounts of fluid and how long it takes until they re-equilibrate and can be functional again, only to fall into the same cycle of misery every other day. However, unphysiological fluid removal is not the only factor implicated in our failure as nephrologists to alleviate our patients' predicaments.

After the inception of dialysis, the thinking, erroneous as it might now be perceived as, was that more efficient machines would allow us to shorten the dialysis time since, supposedly, higher clearances of small solutes would improve outcomes. This is not necessarily so. The HEMO study has shown that increasing predialysis concentration of serum β2 microglobulin (β2M), a known marker of larger solutes accumulated in uremic patients, is a primary risk factor for mortality in ESRD.[16] In addition, it is currently recognized that removal of larger solutes, commonly designated as "middle molecules," requires a longer dialysis time and convective mass transfer across the dialyzer membrane in order to reduce elevated levels of β2M.[17–21]

Besides, it stands to reason that particles of different molecular weight will move at different speeds when subjected to equal kinetic forces. The larger the molecule, the slower it moves, therefore requiring more time to transit any given distance. As a result, removal of middle molecules necessitates longer dialysis duration to accomplish their removal. Also, the main volume of distribution of middle molecules is intracellular, therefore requiring a longer time to move from the intracellular to the interstitial space and from there to the vascular space from which they can be removed with dialysis. Convective transport has been suggested as a more effective tool than diffusion for the removal of these molecules from ESRD patients.[18–21]

Numerous compounds identified as potentially toxic when accumulated in uremic patients[22] are accumulated mostly in the protein-bound form, while the free form found in plasma seems to be responsible for their toxicity. As the protein-free fraction may be amenable to removal by dialysis or hemodiafiltration, as soon as the treatment is completed the protein-bound form will re-equilibrate, with the protein-free fraction restoring the toxic plasma levels. Therefore, prolonged removal of these toxins by a significant increase in the dialysis time may be the only way to keep the free form of these compounds at a normal level. Of course, this hypothesis, sensible as it may be, has yet to undergo the rigors of clinical trials to prove its validity.

Phosphate is another independent factor of all causes of mortality in ESRD.[11] The majority of the phosphate is not stored in the plasma but in the intracellular space and it cannot be efficiently removed from patients on dialysis unless enough time is allowed for the excess phosphate to transit from the intracellular to the interstitial fluid and from there to the vascular space until it is finally removed by the dialyzer.[23–26]

So far all these data suggest that prolonged dialysis time and increased frequency of treatment may offer the best chance of alleviating the suffering and increasing the longevity of ESRD patients.

On the other hand, implementation of daily dialysis as the standard of care, desirable as it may seem, encounters insurmountable obstacles that make its widespread adoption almost impossible to achieve for the vast majority of ESRD patients.[2,3,27–31] If daily dialysis were to be delivered in the dialysis units, the required capital to build the additional capacity to deliver this amount of care would simply not be available in any country of the world. There are no funds in sight to pay for the additional treatments, nor are there enough technicians and nurses to deliver additional care. Most patients are unlikely to accept additional hours in a bed or an armchair hooked up to the big machine while being unable to conduct other activities of daily life. Even though a small minority of ESRD patients are willing to train themselves as well as friends and families, to perform treatments in their home, the vast majority of them are unable or unwilling to do so.

Consequently, it is incumbent upon nephrologists worldwide to come up with creative ways of delivering more dialysis time, more frequently and more effectively, to more and more patients at a lower cost and utilizing fewer resources. Although these are no small tasks, the plight and mortality of the ESRD patients leave the nephrology community no other alternative.[32]

It is abundantly clear that miniaturized devices that can be worn or implanted on the patient's body are the most likely solution to the problem. Although for decades the development of wearable devices has been the holy grail pursued by many,[33-39] most attempts failed to reach widespread application, mainly because they did not have access to adequate power sources such as the light and small batteries available today, biocompatible and light plastic materials, and advanced electronics. Poorly performing membranes and incomplete understanding of the role of convective transport in the efficiency of mass transfer across the dialyzer membrane were also impediments to producing a miniaturized device that would replace the large and cumbersome machine we still use.

As daily dialysis emerged as a possible better therapy for ESRD patients, the race to miniaturize the dialysis machine as we know it acquired new impetus. Several groups have emerged with new thinking on how to accomplish the task of creating smaller devices that will disrupt the current constraints mentioned above and deliver more dialysis time, preferably in a continuous fashion.

Wearable devices based on the use of the peritoneum as a filter have been advocated by at least three different groups.[40-42] Although the idea of using the peritoneum as a filter is a time-honored one, only one group has ever published animal data[40] and there is a dearth of data in either animals or humans on the actual implementation of such a technology. The main advantage of using the peritoneum as part of a wearable device is the avoidance of heparin or other anticoagulation, since no blood ever circulates through the device. The problems with this type of device are the need to employ the same glucose hypertonic solutions used currently to control fluid overload in any other peritoneal dialysis technique and the potential loss of filtrating capacity by the peritoneum. In addition, we still have not seen the delivery of clearances that would make such devices adequate options for RRT. Yet, it is reasonable to expect that as further research is pursued in this direction a workable device may emerge that will provide one more alternative to currently used technologies.

Several other researchers have embarked on harnessing nanotechnology to develop alternative RRT miniaturized devices. The "human

nephron filter"[43,44] is a proposed device that consists of two membranes operating in series, with the purpose of mimicking the
glomerular filtration with the first membrane and the tubular reab-
sorption of water and solutes with the second membrane. The
membrane pores are designed and constructed to allow convective
transport and selective filtration of molecules up to a desired size,
and the pores in the second membrane are designed to reject, by
being electrically charged, undesirable solutes, which are therefore
excreted whilst allowing other solutes (i.e. sodium and calcium) and
water to be reabsorbed. Bicarbonate supplementation may be
required. Since this model does not require dialysate or large energy
sources, it is conceivable that its implementation will generate a very
smart and elegant solution to the need for miniaturized RRT devices.
The device assumes a blood flow of 100 ml/min and a urea clearance
of 62 ml/min. On the other hand, it is unclear how fluids would be
propelled through this device or how water removal from the body
would be accomplished from filtration to a fluid collection bag. Also,
how to overcome the challenge of anticoagulation requirements with
the proposed apparatus is unclear. The device has undergone virtual
simulation which suggests that it is feasible but there are no actual
data published on the performance of the device on bench proto-
types or animals. However, this is an elegant and praiseworthy
proposition which, if given adequate support, may result in insignifi-
cant advances in this field.

Similarly, other authors[45] have initiated the development of
miniaturized and highly efficient membranes based on the principle
that slit shaped nanopores 10–100 nm × 45 mm may have superior
filtration capabilities as compared to cylindrical or convoluted pores
of currently used polymer-based membranes.[46] Micromachined and
microfabricated membranes utilizing microelectromechanic
techniques (MEMS) using silicone oxide (with covalent polyethylene
glycol surface modification) were tested. Since silicon-based
membranes are potent activators of the coagulation cascade, the
novelty of this modification conferring additional biocompatibility
on these membranes is a significant step in the development of this
approach. From this step to a viable RRT device is a lengthy, arduous

and challenging path. The construction and testing of a working RRT prototype using these membranes is yet to be accomplished. However, the promise of this development is attractive and hopefully one day it may result in a paradigm shift in the way RRT is delivered.

Dialysis between two flowing, miscible fluids without an intervening membrane enhances both the transport rate and the biocompatibility.[47,48] Stable flows of one fluid sheathing another miscible fluid are achievable and molecular exchange between the fluids is orderly and in qualitative agreement with the theory. Therefore, "membraneless dialysis" has been proposed as a mechanism for diffusive interchange. However, this concept would still require a pump and a small dialyzer to complete efficient RRT. Although currently there are no bench or animal data available on any RRT prototype built or tested based on this concept, this approach remains for now a meritorious idea that may deliver significant advances in the quest for miniaturized RRT devices.

Current RRT in ARF only substitutes for the filtration function of the kidney, and but not its cellular metabolic functions. Replacing these metabolic functions may optimize current therapy for this devastating disease process. In this regard, a renal tubule assist device (RAD) has been developed to be placed in an extracorporeal continuous hemoperfusion circuit in series with a conventional hemofilter. The use of live tubular cells grown in the laboratory, and incorporated into conventional dialyzers, has resulted in the construction of a bioartificial kidney.[49-51] Available data indicate that this therapy holds the promise of significant improvement in the outcomes of acute kidney injury and multiorgan failure.[51] The most important discovery in this technique is the previously unappreciated role of tubular cells in recovery from catastrophic sepsis, acute kidney injury and multiorgan failure. The application of these fundamental achievements to the treatment of ESRD, although theoretically promising, has not been shown to be feasible at this time.

Our team has taken a different approach to producing a better alternative to the current way of treating ESRD. Taking into account that different instruments and machines have undergone significant downsizing and miniaturization, our concept has been to miniaturize the dialysis machine to the point where it will be light, ergonomic and independent of electrical and water sources so that it can be worn on the patient's body. Furthermore, we targeted at building a wearable artificial kidney (WAK) that would deliver continuous renal replacement, very much like the native kidneys filtering our blood 24 h a day.[32] Continuous renal replacement therapy (CRRT) delivers significantly higher doses of dialysis. CRRT machines in their current form are not suitable to be worn by patients on their body. Miniaturizing a CRRT machine was no small undertaking. We were confronted with significant obstacles to our initial development attempts:

(1) We required freedom from the electrical outlet, yet there is a need for enough energy to propel blood and dialysate through the device. This meant that we needed batteries that would be light and still deliver enough power, and we also had to construct highly efficient pumps that would use very little power.

(2) We had to have enough dialysate to achieve satisfactory clearance of the different solutes which we remove from ESRD patients. Since we typically use about 120 l of fresh water to accomplish a regular dialysis treatment, and people could not possibly walk around carrying such a heavy load on themselves, we adopted an already existing sorbent system configured and modified for this specific device but allowing the purification and regeneration of a much smaller amount of dialysate that could be recirculated through the system. Also, there is rising substantiation of the notion that dialysate should be ultrapure and free not only of bacteria but also of toxins and pyrogens. The dialysate circuit of the WAK uses 375 ml of 0.45% normal saline IV fluid, and the tubing and sorbent system are gamma-sterilized, therefore eliminating the problems that may be associated with unsterile, impure or "dirty," toxin-containing dialysate.

(3) In order to drive blood and dialysate through a dialyzer, existing dialysis equipment utilizes two bulky and heavy pumps powered by an electrical cord plugged into an electrical 110 or 220 V outlet. These are peristaltic pumps that generate laminar flow. However, pulsatile flow has been shown to augment convective mass transfer across the filter membrane. In order to implement this concept to improve the efficiency of the system, a unique double channel opposite phase pulsating pump was created. Unlike flow patterns of blood and dialysate with conventional pumps, the WAK pump creates an intermittent oscillating inversion of transmembrane pressures, generating a "push–pull" mechanism that further enhances convective transport (Fig. 1). The pump currently weighs 280 g and is battery-operated. Push–pull mechanisms for increasing convection have been proposed by using a piston pump to propel dialysate[52] but they never were implemented in the market. Similarly, a push–pull pump for propelling blood has been described[53] but no machine [this is the first device ever since the author and colleagues wrote this, somebody has published a

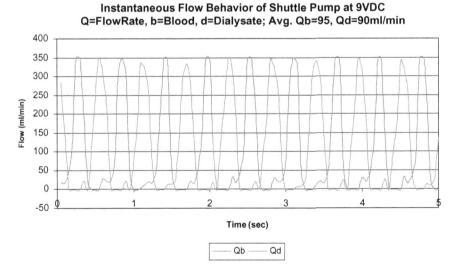

Fig. 1. Shuttle pump flow behavior as described in the text.

double push-pull pattern, but the author's group was first] has ever combined push–pull mechanisms for blood and dialysate. This combination, in opposite phase, has resulted in a single pump that could propel both fluids with less energy whilst performing effective removal of small solutes and middle molecules.[54,55]

(4) The rate of fluid elimination has to be physiological, since it has already been shown that abrupt and excessive ultrafiltration is unphysiological and may result in deleterious effects on ESRD patients. Continuous slow fluid elimination at a rate similar to that performed by native kidneys is accomplished with the WAK keeping patients euvolemic.

(5) The weight, shape and form of the WAK have to allow ergonomic adaptation to the body contour so that it can be worn continuously and permit the patient to sleep, sit and walk comfortably, and even ride in a vehicle or have sex.

(6) Since kidney donors are scarce at best in some parts of the world or nonexistent at worst in several countries, the targeted clearances delivered by the WAK should be similar to those achieved with transplants.

The use of REDY sorbents in initial attempts to build a WAK has not come to fruition yet. REDY sorbent cartridges weigh about 2.27 kg and are not ergonomically suitable for a wearable device. We modified and configured the REDY system to make it light and ergonomically appropriate for a WAK. The initial prototype WAK, worn as a belt, weighed about 10 lb and was initially tried on the bench in our laboratory. Subsequently we created an animal model of kidney failure in pigs and showed the initial evidence of the safety and efficacy of the WAK in animals.[52] Like any other CRRT machine, the WAK can be used for ultrafiltration in the treatment of fluid overload.[58] This use is specifically relevant to the treatment of NYH class III and IV congestive heart failure.[58,59] In fluid-overloaded animals the device achieved fluid removal of up to 700 ml per hour with no difficulties. In six human subjects ultrafiltration was conducted safely and efficiently and no untoward effects were detected.

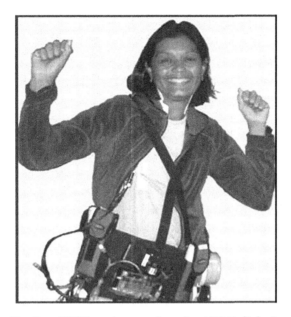

Fig. 2.   ESRD patient undergoing WAK dialysis.

Then, another pilot human study with the WAK was undertaken over eight humans for periods varying between 4 and 8 h (Fig. 2).[55] All participants in this trial tolerated the treatment with the WAK. None complained of any symptoms or developed any complications. Patients had no difficulties sleeping, walking, sitting, eating or drinking. Urea clearance was 22.7 ± 5.2 and creatinine clearance was 20.7 ± 4.8 ml/min. Hourly kt/v was 0.035. The average hourly amount of β2 microglobulin removed was 15.59 ± 9.86 mg/h (1.32 ± 0.84 umol/h), with a β2 microglobulin clearance of 11.3 ± 2.3 ml/min. The average amount of phosphate removed was 445.2 ± 325.9 mg at a mean hourly rate of 69.56 mg/h ± 50.92 (2.24 ± 1.64 mmol/h), with a plasma phosphorus clearance of 21.7 ± 4.5 ml/min.[61]

These data are consistent with our previous *in vitro* laboratory studies, which showed that the pulsatile blood/dialysate pump produced a push–pull type of hemodiafiltration, effectively removing β2 microglobulin from normal blood, as nearly all of the β2 microglobulin cleared into the dialysate was adsorbed by the sorbents.[62]

The WAK is now beyond feasibility and proof of concept both in animal models and in human subjects. Further clinical trials will be needed to determine its real impact on reducing cost and the use of resources, and, more importantly, on improving morbidity and mortality in ESRD patients.

Sterile dialysate will contribute to eliminating real or perceived difficulties ascribed to the current use of "dirty" water which is not free of bacterial toxins. That the WAK uses only 375 ml of sterile fluid makes the use of the highest quality fluid cost-effective. The WAK is intended for continuous use, 24 h a day, 7 days a week — about 16 times more treatment hours than with the standard 3-weekly treatments. On the other hand, it will give patients much more freedom to conduct normal activities of daily life. Hopefully it will allow many of them to become working taxpayers, as opposed to being disabled welfare recipients. As data from daily intermittent dialysis studies already suggest, significant cost savings are to be expected from reduced hospitalizations and drug consumption. In addition, it is reasonable to expect additional savings from the reduction in nursing and technical labor necessary for delivering dialysis today.

Significant improvements in patients' quality of life might be achieved as water, salt, potassium and phosphorus are removed continuously in a slow and effective manner, therefore eliminating the many draconian dietary restrictions we impose on these unfortunate individuals today. The amounts of phosphorus removed by the WAK may get rid of the need for phosphate binders — not only a welcome cost reduction but also definite relief from the "pill burden." This would be consistent with data from patients on daily dialysis. Eliminating hyperphosphatemia may result in improvements in renal osteodystrophy, vascular calcifications and secondary hyperparathyroidism. Further prospective studies will be needed to examine these issues.

Upon completion of regulatory approval, the WAK may become the standard of care in dialysis and bring a paradigm change to the way we treat ESRD (Fig. 2).

References

1. US Renal Data System. (2008) http://www.usrds.org
2. Manns BJ, Johnson JA, Taub K, Mortis G, Ghali WA, Donaldson C. (2002) Dialysis adequacy and health-related quality of life in hemodialysis patients. *ASAIO J* **48**: 565–569.
3. Mapes DL, Lopes AA, Satayathum S, McCullough KP, Goodkin DA, Locatelli F, *et al.* (2003) Health-related quality of life as a predictor of mortality and hospitalization: The Dialysis Outcomes and Practice Patterns Study (DOPPS). *Kidney Int* **64**: 339–349.
4. Germain MJ, Cohen LM, Davison SN. Withholding and withdrawal from dialysis: What we know about how our patients die. *Semin Dial* **20**(3): 195–199.
5. Kjellstrand CM, Ing T. (1998) Daily hemodialysis: History and revival of a superior dialysis method. *ASAIO J* **44**: 117–122.
6. Pierratos A. (2002) Daily hemodialysis: An update. *Curr Opin Nephrol Hypertens* **11**: 165–171.
7. Lindsay RM, Heidenheim AP, Leitch R, *et al.* (2001) Short daily versus long nocturnal hemodialysis. *ASAIO J* **47**: 449–455.
8. Buoncristiani U, Fagugli R, Quintaliani G, Kulurianu H. (1997) Rationale for daily dialysis. *Home Hemodial Int* **1**: 12–18.
9. Depner T. (1999) Why daily hemodialysis is better: Solute kinetics. *Semin Dial* **12**: 462–471.
10. Pierratos A. (2001) Effect of therapy time and frequency on effective solute removal. *Semin Dial* **14**: 284–288.
11. Chazot C, Jean G. (2009) The advantages and challenges of increasing the duration and frequency of maintenance dialysis sessions. *Nat Clin Pract Nephrol* **5**(1): 34–44.
12. Degoulet P. (1982) Mortality risk factors in patients treated by chronic hemodialysis: Report of the Diaphane collaborative study. *Nephron* **31**: 103–110.
13. Kjellstrand CM, Evans RL, Petersen RJ, Shideman JR, Hartitzsch B, Buselmeier TJ. (2004) The "unphysiology" of dialysis: A major cause of dialysis side effects? *Hemodial Int* **8**(1): 24–29.
14. Movilli E, Gaggia P, Zubani R, Camerini C, Vizzardi V, Parrinello G, *et al.* (2007) Association between high ultrafiltration rates and mortality in

uraemic patients on regular haemodialysis: A 5-year prospective observational multicentre study. *Nephrol Dial Transplant* **22**: 3547–3552.

15. Kimmel PL, Varela MP, Peterson RA, Weihs KL, Simmens SJ, Alleyne S, *et al.* (2000) Interdialytic weight gain and survival in hemodialysis patients: Effects of duration of ESRD and diabetes mellitus. *Kidney Int* **57**(3):1141–1151.

16. Cheung AK, Rocco MV, Yan G, Leypoldt JK, Levin NW, Greene T, *et al.* For HEMO Study Group. (2002) Serum β-2 microglobulin levels predict mortality in dialysis patients: Results of the HEMO study. *J Am Soc Nephrol* **17**: 546–555.

17. Ward RA, Greene T, Hartmann B, Samtleben W. (2006) Resistance to intercompartmental mass transfer limits β2-microglobulin removal by post-dilution hemodiafiltration. *Kidney Int* **69**: 1431–1437.

18. Locatelli FM. Di Filippo S. (2002) The importance of convective transport. *Kidney Int* **80**(*Suppl*): S115–S120.

19. Canaud B, Bragg-Gresham JL, Marshall MR, Desmeules S, Gillespie BW, Depner T, *et al.* (2003) Patients receiving hemofiltration have lower mortality risk than patients receiving hemodialysis without replacement fluid (HD) in Europe: The Dialysis Outcomes and Practice Patterns Study (DOPPS), *J Am Soc Nephrol* **14**: 31A.

20. Jirka T, Cesare S, Di Benedetto A, Perera Chang M, Ponce P, Richards N. (2005) The impact of on-line haemodiafiltration (HDF) on patient survival: Results from a large network database. *Nephrol Dial Transplant* **20**(*Suppl 5*): S18–S19.

21. Raj DSC, Ouwendyk M, Francoeur R, Pierratos A. (2000) β2-microglobulin kinetics in nocturnal haemodialysis. *Nephrol Dial Transplant* **15**: 58–64.

22. Vanholder R, De Smet R, Glorieux G, *et al.* for European Uremic Toxin Work Group (EUTox). (2003) Review on uremic toxins: Classification, concentration, and interindividual variability. *Kidney Int* **63**: 1934–1943.

23. Young EW, Akiba T, Albert JM, McCarthy JT, Kerr PG, Mendelssohn DC, Jadoul M. (2004) Magnitude and impact of abnormal mineral metabolism in hemodialysis patients in the Dialysis Outcomes and Practice Patterns Study (DOPPS). *Am J Kidney Dis* **44**(*Suppl 3*): 34–38.

24. Zehnder C, Gutzwiller JP, Renggli K. (1999) Hemodiafiltration — a new treatment option for hyperphosphatemia in hemodialysis patients. *Clin Nephrol* **52**: 152–159.

25. Albalate C, Fernandez MD, Lopez C, Cago A, Jarraiz A, Pulido A, *et al.* (2003) Can we increase phosphate removal with conventional hemodialysis? *Nefrologia* **23**: 520–527.

26. Gutzwiller JP, Schneiditz D, Huber AR, Schindler E, Zehnder CE. (2003) Increasing blood flow increases kt/V (urea) and potassium removal but fails to improve phosphate removal. *Clinic Nephrol* **59**: 130–136.

27. Lockridge Jr RS. (2004) The direction of end-stage renal disease reimbursement in the United States. *Semin Dial* **17**: 125–130.

28. Lockridge Jr RS, McKinney JK. (2001) Is HCFA's reimbursement policy controlling quality of care for end-stage renal disease patients? *ASAIO J* **47**: 466–468.

29. McFarlane PA, Bayoumi AM, Pierratos A, Redelmeier DA. (2003) The quality of life and cost utility of home nocturnal and conventional in-center hemodialysis. *Kidney Int* **64**: 1004–1011.

30. Mohr PE, Neumann PJ, Franco SJ, Marainen J, Lockridge R, Ting G. (2001) The case for daily dialysis: Its impact on costs and quality of life. *Am J Kidney Dis* **37**: 777–789.

31. Patel SS, Shah VS, Peterson RA, Kimmel PL. (2002) Psychosocial variables, quality of life, and religious beliefs in ESRD patients treated with hemodialysis. *Am J Kidney Dis* **40**: 1013–1022.

32. Gura V, Ronco C, Davenport A. (2009) The wearable artificial kidney, why and how: From holy grail to reality. *Semin Dial* **22**(1): 13–17.

33. Beltz AD. Inventor: Wearable, portable, light-weight artificial kidney. US patent 5284470, 2/8/1994.

34. Bonomini V, Roggeri G. Inventors: Hemodialysis and/or ultrafiltration apparatus. US patent 4269708, 5/26/1981.

35. Kolff WJ, Jacobsen S, Stephen RL, Rose D. (1976) Towards a wearable artificial kidney. *Kidney Int (Suppl 7)*: S300–S304.

36. Mineshima M. (2004) Artificial kidney therapy in next generation. *Nippon Rinsho* **62**(*Suppl 6*): 606–609.

37. Shaldon S, Beau MC, Deschodt G, Lysaght MJ, Ramperez P, Mion C. (1980) Continuous ambulatory hemofiltration. *Trans Am Soc Artif Intern Organs* **26**: 210–223.

38. Murisasco A, Reynier JP, Ragon A, Boobes Y, Baz M, Durand C, *et al.* (1986) Continuous arterio-venous hemofiltration in a wearable device

to treat end-stage renal disease. *Trans Am Soc Artif Intern Organs* **32**: 567–571.

39. Senoo S, Otsubo O, Watanabe T, Yamauchi J, Yamada Y, Inou T, *et al.* (1982) The wearable artificial kidney: Development of a small blood pump. *Jinkou Zouki* **11**: 48.

40. Lee DB, Roberts M. (2008) A peritoneal-based automated wearable artificial kidney. *Clin Exp Nephrol* **12**(3): 171–180.

41. Ronco C, Fecondini L. The Vicenza wearable artificial kidney for peritoneal dialysis (ViWAK PD). (2007) *Blood Purif* **25**(4): 383–388.

42. Ofsthun NJ. Personal communication.

43. Nissenson AR, Ronco C, Pergamit G, Edelstein M, Watts R. (2005) Continuously functioning artificial nephron system: The promise of nanotechnology. *Hemodial Int* **9**(3): 210–217.

44. Nissenson AR, Ronco C, Pergamit G, Edelstein M, Watts R. (2005) The human nephron filter: Toward a continuously functioning, implantable artificial nephron system. *Blood Purif* **23**(4): 269–274.

45. Fissell WH, Dubnisheva A, Eldridge AN. (2009) High performance silicon nanopore hemofiltration membranes. *J Membr Sci* **326**: 58–63.

46. Ronco C, Bowry S. (2001) Nanoscale modulation of the pore dimensions, size distribution and structure of a new polysulfone-based high-flux dialysis membrane. *Int J Artif Organs* **24**: 726–735.

47. Leonard EF, Cortell S, Vitale NG. (2005) Membraneless dialysis — is it possible? *Contrib Nephrol* **149**: 343–353.

48. Leonard EF, West AC, Shapley NC, Larsen MU. (2004) Dialysis without membranes: How and why? *Blood Purif* **22**(1): 92–100.

49. Fissell WH, Manley S, Westover A, Humes HD, Fleischman AJ, Roy S. (2006) Differentiated growth of human renal tubule cells on thin-film and nanostructured materials. *ASAIO J.* **52**(3): 221–227.

50. Ding F, Humes HD. (2008) The bioartificial kidney and bioengineered membranes in acute kidney injury. *Nephron Exp Nephrol* **109**(4): e118–e122.

51. Tiranathanagul K, Brodie J, Humes HD. (2006) Bioartificial kidney in the treatment of acute renal failure associated with sepsis. *Nephrology (Carlton)* **11**(4): 285–291.

52. Gura V, Beizai M, Ezon C, Polaschegg HD. (2005) The wearable artificial kidney (WAK). *Contrib Nephrol* **149**: 325–333.

53. Shinzato T, Maeda K. (2007) Push/pull hemodiafiltration. *Contrib Nephrol* **158**: 169–176.
54. Ash SR. (2004) The Allient dialysis system. *Semin Dial* **17**(2): 164–166.
55. Davenport A, Gura V, Ronco C, Beizai M, Ezon C, Rambod E. (2007) A wearable haemodialysis device for patients with end-stage renal failure: A pilot study. *Lancet* **370**: 2005–2010.
56. Gura V, Davenport A, Beizai M, Ezon C, Ronco C. (2009) Beta(2)-microglobulin and phosphate clearances using a wearable artificial kidney: A pilot study. *Am J Kidney Dis*.
57. Ronco C, Davenport A, Gura V. (2008) A wearable artificial kidney: Dream or reality? *Nat Clin Pract Nephrol* **4**(11): 604–605.
58. Gura V, Beizai M, Ezon C, Rambod E. (2006) Continuous renal replacement therapy for congestive heart failure: The wearable continuous ultrafiltration system. *ASAIO J* **52**(1): 59–61.
59. Gura V, Ronco C, Nalesso F, Brendolan A, Beizai M, Ezon C, *et al.* (2008) A wearable hemofilter for continuous ambulatory ultrafiltration. *Kidney Int* **73**(4): 497–502.
60. Gura V, Davenport A, Beizai M, Ezon C, Ronco C. (2009) Beta(2)-microglobulin and phosphate clearances using a wearable artificial kidney: A pilot study. *Am J Kidney Dis*.
61. Gura V, Beizai M, Ezon C, Snukal R, Rambod E. (2006) The wearable artificial kidney (WAK) removes beta2-microglobulins (B2M). *J Am Soc Nephrol* **17**: 723A–724A.
62. Chiu YW, Teitelbaum I, Misra M, de Leon EM, Adzize T, Mehrotra R. (2009) Pill burden, adherence, hyperphosphatemia, and quality of life in maintenance dialysis patients. *Clin J Am Soc Nephrol*.

CHAPTER 10

Xenotransplantation

Moro O. Salifu,[*,†] Syed Shah[†] and Subodh Saggi[†]*

Following the first successful syngraft (identical twin–twin kidney transplantation) in 1955,[1] this therapy has been extended to include different types of allografts (nontwin human–human transplantation) from living and deceased donors. The increasing prevalence of end stage renal disease (ESRD)[2] as well as many other vital organ failures but grossly insufficient number of allografts calls for novel ways, notably xenografts (organs or tissues from different species), to meet this ever-increasing demand. Currently 13 patients die each day in the United States while on the waiting list to receive life-saving vital organ transplants and about 60% of patients with organ failure die without ever receiving a transplant. In this chapter, we will review the concept of xenotransplantation and some of the challenges that need to be met before clinical xenotransplantation becomes a reality.

The Concept of Xenotransplantation

The United Sates Public Health Service (USPHS) and the Food and Drug Administration (FDA)[3,4] define xenotransplantation ("xeno-" is from the Greek word meaning "foreign") as any procedure that involves the transplantation, implantation, or infusion into a human recipient of either (1) live cells, tissues, or organs from a nonhuman animal source or (2) human body fluids, cells, tissues or organs that

*Corresponding author.
[†]Division of Nephrology, SUNY Downstate Medical Center Brooklyn, New York, USA.
Email: moro.salifu@downstate.edu

Table 1.   Animal Tissues and Organs Considered for Xenotransplantation

Donor Source	Tissues/Cells and Organs for Xenotransplantation
Chimpanzee	Kidney[21]
Baboon	Heart,[22] liver,[23] bone marrow[24]
Pig	Liver,[25] Heart valves[26,27] pancreatic islet cells,[28] Neural cells,[29] skin graft,[30,31]
Cow	Adrenal (chromaffin) cells[32]
Goat	Heart valves,[33] hepatocytes[34]
Fish (shark)	Spinal cord cells[35]

have had *ex vivo* contact with live nonhuman animal cells, tissues, or organs. These live cells, tissues, or organs used in xenotransplantation are considered products by the FDA.

Table 1 summarizes different types of animal cells, tissue, and organs considered for xenotransplantation. While xenotransplantation remains largely experimental, especially for solid organ (kidney, liver, heart, and pancreas) transplantation, and is heavily regulated by the FDA, there have been successes in the application of xenotransplantation for certain human diseases. For example, direct implantation of animal cells, tissues, and organs has been accomplished in nonhuman bone marrow cells for human transplantation, nonhuman neuronal cells for Parkinson's disease, and nonhuman liver cells for human liver transplantation. In some diseases, involving for example pancreatic islet cells for restoring insulin production in diabetic patients or neuronal cells for treating neurodegenerative disease, human materials are not usually available and animals are the only source.

Whatever the source, the primary goal of xenotransplantation is restoration of the human physiologic state, physical functioning, and prolonged survival. The success of xenotransplantation will greatly eliminate the need to be on the wait list for tissue or organ transplantation and ensure that certain vital organ failures as well as nonvital but disabling chronic diseases are cured by replacement. Despite these benefits, xenotransplantation remains largely experimental, with safety and efficacy concerns. Several barriers must be crossed before this therapy can gain widespread acceptance and use. Even when it survives, it is unclear if the physiologic function of xenografts will mirror that required for human physiologic function as proteins produced by xenografts may not necessarily have the same physiologic effects in humans.[5]

Immunologic Barriers

The immune system is designed to distinguish self from nonself antigens. The genes responsible for this recognition are collectively known as major histocompatibility complex (MHC) genes. In humans, MHC gene products are called human leucocyte antigens (HLAs), located on various cell surfaces. When nonself antigens are encountered, the immune system is activated through the HLA system, mounting various types of reactions involving humoral and cellular mechanisms of rejection. It follows then that the closer the immune system is between donor and recipient, the less likely rejection will be. As a result, autografts (transplantation of tissue from one part of the body to another in the same individual) and syngrafts (identical twin–twin transplantation) eliminate the need to suppress the immune system. Outside these, immunosuppression is the norm. At least within the same species as in allotransplantation, antigenic differences cannot be as large as will be encountered when one is transplanting between animals and humans, and therefore xenotransplantation raises serious immunologic concerns.[6] Furthermore, testing of the HLA system has aided risk stratification of human transplantation, but it is unclear which system of antigenic testing will be used to determine compatibility between animal antigens (xenoantigens) and human antigens (alloantigens). Thus, much is yet to be done in defining xenoantigen testing and its impact on rejection. Some of the potential immunologic responses to xenotransplantation are:

Hyperacute rejection. This is defined as rejection of the xenograft within minutes to hours after implantation. It is mediated by naturally occurring antibodies in humans that do not recognize xenoantigens and therefore bind to them activating complement.[7] The membrane attack complex, a final byproduct of complement activation, destroys endothelial and other cellular components, resulting in destruction of the xenograft.[8] The larger the phylogenic distance between the species, the stronger the reaction, as shown by better acceptance between humans and other primates compared with human–pig xenotransplantation.[9]

Delayed xenograft rejection. This is defined as rejection of the xenograft within days to months after implantation. The mechanism of delayed rejection is poorly understood but is also connected with naturally occurring antibodies in humans that do not recognize xenoantigens and therefore bind to them activating complement, resulting in rejection but at a slower rate than for hyperacute rejection.[10]

Cellular xenograft rejection: Xenografts that survive both hyperacute and delayed rejection may still encounter cellular rejection mediated by lymphocyte and other cellular activation.[11]

Improving Xenograft Survival

Immunosuppression. Since hyperacute and delayed xenograft rejection are mediated for the most part by circulating antibodies, immunosuppression will have little impact. The effect of reducing circulating antibodies[12] and the use of complement inhibitors such as soluble complement receptors prior to xenotransplantation, are promising, although many challenges remain. Thus, the main target of immunosuppression, at least in animal studies, has been to suppress the cellular arm of the reaction. This strategy has been shown to be possible using conventional immunosuppression,[13] although no studies on humans exist to confirm these observations.

Genetic engineering. If the xenograft can be altered to express human complement regulatory proteins, as in the case of transgenically engineered pigs,[14] or reduce the expression of key proteins such as the alpha-Gal epitope, the main pig antigen recognized by the human immune system,[15] then xenografts may be better accommodated and the chance of rejection significantly reduced.

Application of physical barriers. To avoid immunologic attack when animal cells are administered through the human bloodstream, methods such as encapsulation, as in pancreatic islet cell transfer,[16] or via semipermeable membranes, as in the treatment of severe liver failure using a porcine bioartificial liver,[17] are under development and remain largely experimental.

Infectious Barriers

Transmission of infectious disease from xenografts to humans (zoonosis) has been the most serious concern in clinical xenotransplantation. This concern is supported by the fact that even in allotransplantation infectious agents such as HIV and hepatitis viruses can be transmitted from human to human. Not only is it a concern for the recipient, but is also a major concern that the general population may be exposed to a previously unidentified infection, leading to an epidemic.[18] Furthermore, screening tests for infectious agents using current serologic and microbiologic culture techniques are available only for known infectious agents. The broader concern is detection of new or emerging infections that may not necessarily cause human disease under natural conditions, but may become infectious or pathogenic after xenotransplantation. Table 2 lists some of the known zoonostic infections after transplantation.

Ethical Issues

The lack of answers to many of the questions regarding xenotransplantation, particularly those related to rejection and infectious agents, raises serious concerns about informed consent and privacy of medical information. Patients must understand that risks are also public health risks and that privacy may be compromised. They should be made aware of the need for isolation, travel limitations, and lifetime surveillance.[19] Animals have different lifespans than humans and

Table 2.   Infections Associated with Xenotransplantation

Viral Infections

Exogenous viruses[36,37]
    Porcine hepatitis E virus
    Circoviruses
    Paramyxoviruses
    Orthomyxoviruses
    Parvoviruses
    Porcine gammaherpesviruses
    Porcine lymphotropic herpesvirus (PLHV)
    Porcine cytomegalovirus (PCMV)
    Baboon cytomegalovirus (BCMV)[38]

Endogenous viruses
    Porcine endogenous retrovirus (PERV), types A, B, and C[36,37]
    Baboon endogenous retrovirus (BaEV)[39]

Bacterial infections[18]
    Conventional bacterial infections associated with immunosuppression

Fungal infections[18]
    Conventional fungal infections associated with immunosuppression

Others
    Unknown emerging infections

their tissues age at a different rate, raising more questions than answers. Further, there is the concern that animals are used for human benefit and whether this approach is ethical. Disease transmission and permanent alteration to the genetic code of humans are also cause for concern. Is it ethical for an individual to affect negatively the whole human population as a result of a single decision? These and many more ethical questions retard the clinical application of xenotransplantation, and until such questions are properly answered its future remains uncertain.

Conclusion

Although xenotransplantation is at the cutting edge of medical science and can potentially save thousands of lives, it has deeper implications that extend beyond the realm of the individual in organ or system failure into a social dimension that makes ethical acceptability even more difficult. To gain a rational perspective on the ethical, moral, and social issues provoked by a contemplated specific xenotransplantation, the preparatory discussion must include all stakeholders as well as pertinent regulatory agencies globally involved in safeguarding health. Ethical and legal standards must be designed to balance concern over potential epidemics due to transmitted animal infections such as the Ebola virus infection which followed handling of infected African chimpanzees, gorillas, and antelopes,[20] while facilitating clinical trials of experimental xenotransplants that may alleviate an ever-increasing organ shortage.

References

1. Guild WR, Harrison JH, Merrill JP, Murray J. (1955) Successful homo-transplantation of the kidney in an identical twin. *Trans Am Clin Climatol Assoc* **67**: 167–173.

2. US Renal Data System. (2008) USRDS 2008 Annual Data Report: Atlas of Chronic Kidney Disease and End-Stage Renal Disease in the United States. National Institutes of Health, National Institute of Diabetes and Digestive and Kidney Diseases (Bethesda, MD).

3. PHS Guideline on Infectious Disease Issues in Xenotransplantation (USPHS, Jan 19, 2001). Available at http://www.fda.gov/cber/guidelines. htm, accessed Jun 27, 2009.

4. Draft Guidance for Industry: Precautionary Measures to Reduce the Possible Risk of Transmission of Zoonoses by Blood and Blood Products from Xenotransplantation Product Recipients and Their Contacts. (FDA, Dec 23, 1999). Available at http://www.fda.gov/cber/guidelines. htm, accessed Jun 27, 2009.

5. Lawson JH, Daniels LJ, Platt JL. (1998) The evaluation of thrombomodulin activity in porcine to human xenotransplantation. *Transplant Proc* **29**: 884–885.

6. Auchincloss Jr H, Sachs DH. (1998) Xenogeneic transplantation. *Annu Rev Immunol* **16**: 433–470.

7. Samuelsson BE, Rydberg L, Breimer ME, *et al.* (1994) Natural antibodies and human xenotransplantation. *Immunol Rev* **141**: 151–168.

8. Wang H, DeVries M, Deng S, *et al.* (2000) The axis of interleukin 12 and gamma interferon regulates acute vascular xenogeneic rejection. *Nat Med* **6**: 549–554.

9. Parker W, Saadi S, Lin SS, Holzknecht ZE, Bustos M, Platt JL. (1996) Transplantation of discordant xenografts: A challenge revisited. *Immunol Today* **17**: 373–378.

10. Platt JL. (1994) A perspective on xenograft rejection and accommodation. *Immunol Rev* **141**: 127–149.

11. Inverardi L, Pardi R. (1994) Early events in cell-mediated recognition of vascularized xenografts: Cooperative interactions between selected lymphocyte subsets and natural antibodies. *Immunol Rev* **141**: 71–93.

12. Brenner P, Reichenspurner H, Schmoeckel M, *et al.* (2000) Ig-Therasorb immunoapheresis in orthotopic xenotransplantation of baboons with landrace pig hearts. *Transplantation* **69**: 208–214.

13. Johnsson C, Andersson A, Bersztel A, Karlsson-Parra A, Gannedahl G, Tufveson G. (1997) Successful retransplantation of mouse-to-rat cardiac xenografts under immunosuppressive monotherapy with cyclosporine. *Transplantation* **63**: 652–656.

14. Cozzi E, White DJ. (1995) The generation of transgenic pigs as potential organ donors for humans. *Nat Med* **1**: 964–966.

15. Sandrin MS, McKenzie IFC. (1994) Gal alpha(1,3)Gal, the major xenoantigen(s) recognised in pigs by human natural antibodies. *Immunol Rev* **141**: 167–190.

16. Sun Y-L, Ma X, Zhou D, Vacek I, Sun AM. (1993) Porcine pancreatic islets: Isolation, microencapsulation, and xenotransplantation. *Artif Organs* **17**: 727–733.

17. Chen S, Kahaku E, Watanabe F, *et al.* (1997) Treatment of severe liver failure with a bioartificial liver. *Ann N Y Acad Sci* **831**: 350–360.

18. Chapman LE, Folks TM, Salomon DR, Patterson AP, Eggerman TE, Noguchi PD. (1995) Xenotransplantation and xenogeneic infections. *N Engl J Med* **333**: 1498–1501.

19. Vanderpool HY. (1998) Critical ethical issues in clinical trials with xenotransplants. *Lancet* **351**: 1347–1350.

20. Normile D. (2009) Emerging infectious diseases: Scientists puzzle over Ebola-Reston virus in pigs. *Science* **323**: 451.
21. Reemtsma K, McCracken BH, Schlegel JU, *et al.* (1964) Renal hetero-transplantation in man. *Ann Surg* **160**: 384.
22. Bailey LL, Nehlsen-Cannarella SL, Concepcion W, *et al.* (1985) Baboon-to-human cardiac xenotransplantation in a neonate. *JAMA* **254**(23): 3321–3329.
23. Starzl TE, Fung J, Tzakis A, *et al.* (1993) Baboon-to-human liver transplantation. *Lancet* **341**: 65.
24. Michaels MG, Kaufman C, Volberding PA, Gupta P, Switzer WM, Heneine W, *et al.* (2004) Baboon bone-marrow xenotransplant in a patient with advanced HIV disease: Case report and 8-year follow-up. *Transplantation* **78**(11): 1582–1589
25. Chari RS, Collins BH, Magee JC, *et al.* (1994) Brief report: Treatment of hepatic failure with *ex vivo* pig-liver perfusion followed by liver trans-plantation. *N Engl J Med* **331**: 234–237.
26. Stinson EB, Griepp RB, Oyer PE, Shumway NE. (1977) Long-term experience with porcine aortic valve xenografts. *J Thorac Cardiovasc Surg* **73**(1): 54–63.
27. Fann JI, Miller DC, Moore KA, Mitchell RS, Oyer PE, Stinson EB, *et al.* (1996) Twenty-year clinical experience with porcine bioprostheses. *Ann Thorac Surg* **62**(5): 1301–1311; discussion 1311–1312.
28. Rood PP, Cooper DK. (2006) Islet xenotransplantation: Are we really ready for clinical trials? *Am J Transplant* **6**(6): 1269–1274.
29. Fink JS, Schumacher JM, Ellias SL, *et al.* (2000) Porcine xenografts in Parkinson's disease and Huntington's disease patients: Preliminary results. *Cell Transplant* **9**(2): 273–278.
30. Chiu T, Burd A. (2005) Xenograft dressing in the treatment of burns. *Clin Dermatol* **23**(4): 419–423.
31. Chatterjee DS. (1978) A controlled comparative study of the use of porcine xenograft in the treatment of partial thickness skin loss in an occupational health centre. *Curr Med Res Opin* **5**(9): 726–733.
32. Cooper DKC, Lanza RP. (2000) *Xeno: The Promise of Transplanting Animal Organs into Humans.* Oxford University Press, New York.
33. Yang SS, Maranhao V, Ablaza SG, Morse DP, Nichols HT, Goldberg H. (1969) Clinical and hemodynamic findings following calf aortic valve

transplantation for human aortic valve: A preliminary report. *Am J Cardiol* **23**(2): 199–207.

34. Jayaraman KS. (2003) Goats to deliver cells for transplants in India. *Nat Med* **9**: 491–491.

35. Guidelines for Xenotransplantation. (2003) Correspondence. **349**(13): 1294–1295.

36. Patience, C, Stoye, J. (2004) Infectious risk of clinical xenotransplantation. *Curr Opin Organ Transplant* **9**: 176.

37. Fishman JA, Patience C. (2004) Xenotransplantation: Infectious risk revisited. *Am J Transplant* **4**(9): 1383–1390.

38. Teotia, Sumeet S, Christopher GA, *et al.* (2005) Prevention, detection, and management of early bacterial and fungal infections in a preclinical cardiac xenotransplantation model that achieves prolonged survival. *Xenotransplantation* **12**(2): 127–133.

CHAPTER 11

Can the Bowel Serve as a Kidney?

*Eli A. Friedman**

By the turn of the last century, the quest for replacement of failed vital organs successfully stimulated implantation of artificial hearts, ventricular assist devices, and primitive artificial ears and eyes, as well as gave rise to the novel concept of performing solute extraction from the blood of uremic individuals by having them wear an artificial kidney. In the 21st century, we struggle to relieve a form of conceptual maturation arrest imposed by the realization that the high cost of bionic innovation limits its application for the majority of nations. In fact, as clinically practiced, neither hemodialysis nor peritoneal dialysis has shown any substantial evolution over the past decade. Artificial heart deployment is currently minimal though the device has undergone incremental improvements. Long-term artificial lungs remain an unrealized concept.

Willem J. Kolff, the inventor of the artificial kidney, like the majority of artificial organ enthusiasts, speaking at the 1964 inauguration of the European Dialysis and Transplant Association (EDTA), in a talk entitled: "To Live Without Heart and Kidneys," ebulliently predicted that: "The symbol of life, the site of love, and the habitat of the soul, the human heart, will be replaced by a mechanical pump."[1] Having lived through the transformation of irreversible kidney failure from a death sentence to a treatable disorder, it was easy for one to believe that medical practice was "just around the corner from implantable self-sensing insulin pumps, artificial livers, and an implantable kidney."[2]

*Downstate Medical Center, 450 Clarkson Avenue, Brooklyn, New York 11203, USA.
Email: Elifriedman@aol.com

The "doctor's office" was about to be transformed into a repair shop providing spare part replacement. Little attention was devoted to dealing with the cost of onrushing medical magic because many thought that with American mass production (history's greatest war having been won), America should be able to quickly reduce per patient expense to a negligible amount. Nephrologists thought that industrialized nations would extend renal replacement therapy, with its cost expected to be sharply decreased, to less wealthy nations making death in uremia a rarity.

History, however, records a different global reaction to the new means of averting death in kidney failure. For example, the EDTA, in 1980, analyzed 14,084 incident patients with end-stage renal disease (ESRD) in 32 European countries, noting that of 3786 who received a kidney transplant[3] there was a strong linkage between the rate per million population treated for ESRD in 35 countries and the per capita gross national product in dollars. The disparity between affluent nations able to proffer ESRD care at a rate in excess of 200 per million (Japan, US, Switzerland), and poor nations unable to rise above 50 per million (South Africa, German Democratic Republic, Greece) was disquieting (Fig. 1). At one extreme, the United Kingdom, a democracy with socialized medicine and no entrepreneurial physician profit from dialysis, ranked near the bottom, with many uremic patients sentenced to an untreated death.[4] Japan, by contrast, a nation devastated by war, permitted dialysis as a private practice business, topped the list. It appeared unlikely, for the foreseeable future, that the world might deliver what health enthusiasts promised.[5]

No resolution to the financial barrier to global extension of uremia therapy had been devised 15 years later,[6] as is the case today[7]: No resolution to the dilemma of death without ESRD therapy for most of the world has been devised. A key inference drawn from cumulative analysis of reports of ESRD therapy, that cost of complex medical care de facto excludes all but the rich, can be validly extended to other organ systems. Death in ESRD like overall mortality is an inverse correlate of each nation's affluence.[8] In a cross-national examination of overall mortality in 25 developed countries, the key correlate of total death rate was each country's gross national product

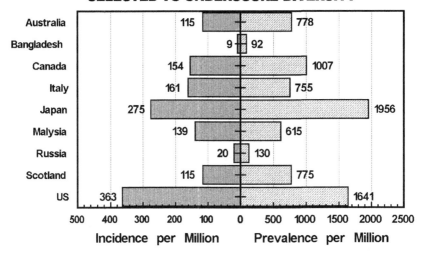

INTERNATIONAL ESRD COMPARISONS
SELECTED TO UNDERSCORE DIVERSITY

USRDS 2008: Data for 2006

Fig. 1. Selected national rates of incidence and prevalence of ESRD therapy as reported in the 2008 report of the United States Renal Data System. The United States and Japan have the highest rates while Bangladesh illustrates the almost total absence of uremia therapy.

(GNP) and not the number of medical doctors, nurses, midwives, or hospital beds; nor was any association detected between total deaths and alcohol or tobacco consumption or military expenditure.[9] After the collapse of communism in Eastern Europe, with relief from low GNP depressed provision of health care[10] dialysis treatment rates tripled.[11] What this means is that even should the restrictions imposed by underfunded national health care systems be removed,[12] for the foreseeable future, there is minimal hope of comprehensive acceptance of present uremia regimens beyond the borders of affluent nations[13] (Figs. 2 and 3).

The challenge for clinical nephrologists is to reduce the cost of treatment for ESRD (a year of hemodialysis requires $40,000 to $80,000 depending on the country) by taking advantage of high technology. A quartz watch that was priced above $3000 when first

OUR TWO WORLDS
ITALY versus CONGO

	ITALY	CONGO
2008 Population	59.9 million	66.5 million
2025 Population	62.0 million	109.7 million
Population below Age 15	8.4 million	31.3 million
Population Age 65 and Older	11.9 million	1.7 million
Annual Births	568,000	2.9 million
Annual Deaths	575,000	843,000
Annual Natural Increase *(births minus deaths)*	-7,000	2.1 million
Annual Infant Deaths	2,300	270,000
Life Expectancy at Birth	**81 years**	**53 years**
Percent of Population Undernourished	< 2.5%	74%

Carl Haub and Mary Mederios Kent, *2008 World Population Data Sheet*

Fig. 2. Illustrative comparison of a relatively wealthy industrialized nation (Italy) and an economically deprived nation (The Congo) in the midst of tribal warfare. Stark contrasts in life expectancy and anticipated population growth through 2025 underscore the impact of economic stress that excludes any probability of universal therapy for ESRD.

introduced, in 2009, today, can be purchased for less than 50 cents. It is not an unreasonable objective to hope for production of bathtubs full of engineered cells programmed to replace failed pancreases, livers, kidneys and lungs. First steps have been taken in the case of substitute kidneys and livers. An additional option for organ replacement was proffered by Chang, over 50 years ago,[14] in the potential design of semi-permeable microcapsules as artificial cells.[15] Artificial cells use ultrathin polymer membrane envelopes, either as spherical membranes containing solutions or suspensions, or as a membrane coating on individual solid granules of adsorbent.[16] Because of their large surface to volume relationship (e.g. 2.5 m^2 surface area in 10 ml of 20 μm diameter or 300 ml of 2–5 mm diameter microcapsules) and their ultrathin membranes (for example, less than 0.05 micron),

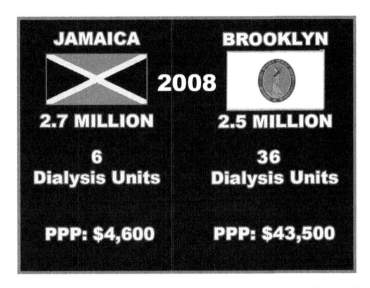

Fig. 3. Comparing the fully industrialized Borough of Brooklyn, in New York City, United States with a purchasing power parity (ppp) of $43,500 in 2008 with an equivalent population, at economic disadvantage in Jamaica with a ppp of $4600 illustrates the impact that economy can impose on delivery of ESRD therapy. Jamaica, in 2008, with 6 small ambulatory hemodialysis units treated ESRD attaining a rate less than 10% that in Brooklyn. Jamaica's ppp in 2008 ranked 93rd of 194 countries according to the Central Intelligence Agency. All less affluent countries had lower rates of ESRD treatment.

artificial cells transport permanent molecules at incredibly rapid rates. Many reports recount the value of oral microencapsulation to replace enzymes in genetic deficiency,[17] as well as of living hepatocytes[18] to control hyperbilirubinemia in the Gunn rat.[19]

Bowel as Kidney

Bowel as a kidney: Oral sorbents

How the intestine may act as a substitute kidney is a fascinating story. The historical and empirical background of a bowel for kidney replacement system have recently been reviewed.[20] Hippocrates vaguely described oral treatment for renal disorders. Use of bowel elimination as a means of managing kidney disease — as reviewed by Thompson[21] — is recorded in Dioscorides Materia Medica in 40 B.C. in which terra sigillata, a sacred earth found on the Greek island of Lemnos, is advocated for multiple disorders including diseases of the kidney. By 100 A.D., Pliny prescribed this esteemed medicine as an oral sorbent against complaints of the spleen and kidneys, copious menstruation, as well as poisons and wounds caused by serpents. Despite the reality that terra sigillata has been forgotten, other oral sorbents including charcoal,[22] oxidized starch,[23] locust bean gum (a mannose polymer derived from seeds of the ceratonia siliqua tree),[24] and microcrystalline carbon with an oxygen complex surface oxide[25] have each been reported in this century as beneficial in the uremic syndrome through promoting nitrogenous waste extraction.

Prior to the introduction of maintenance hemodialysis in 1960, several investigators had documented the potential for nitrogen waste extraction from the human bowel. Schloerb, surgically isolated a loop of ileum and by repeated perfusions with a lactated saline solution was able to prolong the life of otherwise fatally ill young individuals with chronic uremia.[26] Earlier, Willem J. Kolff, inventor of the first practical artificial kidney had speculated on resorting to the gut as a substitute kidney[27] both by lavage (dialysis) and by extraction using an oral sorbent.[28] Sparks had shown that bowel fluid contained sufficient urea, creatinine, and uric acid to suggest that intestinal extraction might be clinically of value[29] by means of ingestion of chemical "binders" now termed sorbents[30]; he had tested a combination of activated charcoal and oxidized starch.

Subsequently, Giordano *et al.*,[31] and later Friedman *et al.*[32] in clinical trials of oxidized starch and charcoal in Naples, Italy and Brooklyn, New York afforded evidence that the bowel might indeed be a useful focus of efforts to remove nitrogenous wastes in uremia. Giordano evaluated the periodic acid oxidation product of starch, dialdehyde starch (oxystarch), as a nitrogen sorbent.[33] Oxystarch under physiologic conditions binds urea at a capacity of 178–277 mmoles/mole of oxystarch aldehyde. After single patient trials, Giordano's team treated cohorts of patients in Naples, Italy with oxystarch at a dose of 30 to 40 g/day for over two years, maintaining a constant blood urea nitrogen concentration, while the serum creatinine gradually rose until the need for dialysis was evident.

AST-120, an oral sorbent comprising particles of porous carbon with a diameter of 0.2 to 0.4 mm, has attracted attention as a means of prolonging the interval until dialytic therapy is mandated. Preliminary studies in Sprague-Dawley rats subjected to 4/5th nephrectomy and then treated with AST-120 1 g/day, revealed delay in onset of glomerular sclerosis while renal function is preserved.[34] Miles *et al.* reported increased mean survival of 7/8ths nephrectomized, AST-120 treated, rats to 104 days as compared with 68 days in controls.[35] Clinical trials, thus far limited to Japan, of AST-120 in a dose of 3.2 to 7.2 g/day to 27 patients with renal insufficiency, prolonged the interval between an azotemic patient's serum creatinine level reaching 6 mg/dl and the start of maintenance hemodialysis, from a mean of 5.0 months in controls to a mean of 14.3 months while improving the severity of anemia. There have been no prospective, double-blind, alternate case evaluation of AST-120 in uremia. In Japan, in 2004, thousands of patients with progressive renal insufficiency were treated with AST 120; Phase 2 studies are in progress in the US.

Diarrhea Therapy

Captain Robert Allan Phillips (1906–1976) as a Navy Lieutenant at the Rockefeller Institute for Medical Research during World War II, devised a field method to assess fluid loss in wounded servicemen, and then embarked on studies during the 1947 Egyptian cholera epidemic that elucidated the pathophysiology of dehydration and death, and devised highly efficacious methods for intravenous fluid repletion.[36] At the United States Naval Medical Research Unit (NAMRU)-2 in Taipei, Phillips conceived of and tested a simple glucose-based oral cholera rehydration therapy to replace the then standard intravenous regimen. Recognizing that as a consequence of profound and sustained diarrhea, those afflicted with cholera evinced a sharp decrease in their plasma levels of nitrogen-containing wastes (urea, creatinine, uric acid), Phillips saw the potential utility of induced diarrhea as a means of treating renal failure. Subsequently, Young *et al.* in Taipei, successfully introduced an oral kidney failure regimen consisting of hyperosmotic fluid containing mannitol 220 mMols/l administered at 240 ml every 5 min until a total of 7 l is reached.[37]

The resulting diarrhea effected a urea clearance of 27.8 ml/min while the bowel creatinine clearance was 7.4 ml/min. Based on a three-hour treatment session, a mean of 4931 mg of non-protein nitrogen was removed, of which 3373 mg was urea nitrogen, during each diarrhea session.[38] Bowel extraction of nitrogen during induced diarrhea is proportional to its initial level in plasma. Chinese uremic patients (creatinine clearance of 2–10 ml/min) were treated in Taipei with thrice weekly induced diarrhea lasting 3–7 hr for up to two years, effecting symptomatic improvement with good tolerance of the regimen. All the patients had improved appetite and less pruritus. When 17 uremic patients practiced diarrhea therapy at home on a thrice-weekly, 3-hr schedule for a mean of 6.8 months with a range of 1.3 to 16 months, a limit was reached when endogenous creatinine clearance fell to 1–2 ml/min, when nausea and vomiting gradually reappeared and signs of fluid retention set in. No objective, controlled, randomized prospective studies of diarrhea therapy as a treatment for advanced kidney failure have been reported. As a consequence, though the concept is appealing, proof of efficacy is lacking. Especially appealing is the low cost of components of the diarrhea regimen which at the time of initial reporting was less than $3.00 per treatment; present costs would be about $9.00 per treatment.

Bacterial enzyme nitrogen recycling within the gut

Ruminant animals are able to utilize cellulose and urea as a source of nutrition because of bacterial metabolism within their intestines[39]; survival for weeks to months following bilateral nephrectomy has been shown in sheep,[40] and cows.[41] Farmers depend on the chemical reactions required when they feed urea and cellulose wastes to cattle which, within the rumen, convert urea to essential amino acids

using cellulose as an energy source. Dairy cows live for six genera-
tions, calve, and produce normal milk on a protein-free diet.[42]
Rumen microbial enzymes by continous exposure to urea and
ammonium salts evolve, gaining the ability to utilize these chemicals
as sole sources of nitrogen permitting protein synthesis. After protein
synthesis within the ruminant animal's gut, digestion and metabolism
of protein following absorption are similar to the processes in non-
ruminant animals.

Setälä, in Helsinki, attempted to emulate ruminant physiology by
administering enzymes extracted from cow feces to uremic patients,
basing the mechanism of his treatments on the hypothesis that bacterial enzymes utilize ammonia, potassium, phosphorus, and other
nitrogenous wastes to cleave vasoconstrictatory peptides in the intestines.[43] Setälä treated 10 uremic patients and 10 normal controls,
with specifically extracted enzymes from cultured (immobilized or
free) "pre-adapted" "apathogenic" soil microorganisms "trained" to
convert urea, creatinine, uric acid, guanidino derivatives, and other
nonprotein nitrogen compounds (NPN) to amino acids utilizing
ammonia, potassium, phosphorus, and other nitrogenous wastes.
During treatment, azotemia and hypertension decreased significantly, only to increase again when the regimen was interrupted.[44]
These studies were interrupted by Setälä's death.

In a reincarnation of the Setälä concept, Prakash and Chang continuously reduced blood urea levels in azotemic rats by instilling
semipermeable microencapsulated genetically engineered live cells
containing living urease-producing *Escherichia coli* DH5.[45]
Previously, these workers demonstrated that genetically engineered
E. coli DH5, contain the urease gene from *K. aerogens* that metabo-
lizes urea without production of ammonia. Pursuing this approach,
bacteria engineered to catabolise unexcreted nitrogenous wastes
within the intestine — termed probiotic bacteria — after being tested
in azotemic rats and miniature pigs, are now being fed in a prospective, double-blind, crossover, placebo-controlled multicenter trial to
patients with CKD.[46] Probiotic bacteria are commonly defined as live
microorganisms, which, when administered in adequate amounts,
confer a health benefit on the host.[47]

Under the clinical trial conducted in an outpatient nephrology clinic in Scarborough, Ontario, Canada, 13 outpatients with CKD Stage 3 or 4 first 3-month treatment period, were randomly assigned to Group A or B and provided capsules containing either placebo or a pro-biotic formulation (90 billion CFU/day, 15 billion/gel cap, 2 caps × 3/day). In the second phase of the study, Groups A and B switched treatment for 3 months. Variables monitored included blood urea nitrogen (BUN), serum creatinine, phosphorus, and uric acid as well as responses to a self-administered quality of life questionnaire. Symptomatic complaints attributed to CKD decreased during administration of probiotic bacteria (Figs. 3 and 4). From this preliminary trial, it appears feasible to expand study of probiotic

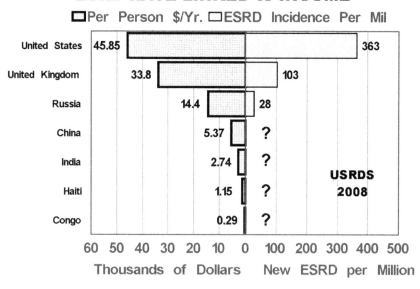

Fig. 4. Comparing, in the left column, purchasing power parity (ppp) of $45,850 in 2008 for the United States and selected populations as listed by the World Bank, with, on the right, the United Kingdom and other countries with ESRD treatment rates too low to register with the United States Renal Data System. This illustrates the author's belief that the world cannot afford contemporary uremia therapy.

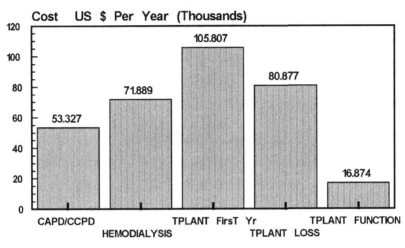

ANNUAL ESRD COST BY MODALITY
US $ Per Year

Cost US $ Per Year (Thousands)

USRDS 2008: Data for 2006

Fig. 5. Considering that the majority of the world's population lives with a family income of less than $1000 per year, facing annual costs of uremia therapy in excess of $50,000 per year, the motivation to devise less expensive therapies is starkly evident. There is hope that specially programmed bacteria, "Probiotics" may be designed such that a low cost oral regimen at a cost of less than $1.00 per day might sustain life after onset of irreversible kidney failure.

formulations as adjunctive health supplements to help stabilize and maintain quality of life in CKD stage 3 and 4 patients. Expanded clinical trials of gut-based probiotic bacteria to determine their value as a component of renoprotection in progressive CKD may assist in sustaining life quality.

An intragut enzyme-based treatment for uremia from a 2009 perspective, is neither novel nor an overly optimistic expression of science fiction. Absent Chang's or other fresh directions in uremia research, our inability to improve the lot of most people with failing kidneys will persist far into this century, resulting in tens of thousands of deaths, very much an outcome of socioeconomic realities. Redefining artificial organs to encompass hybrid devices, smart cells, and even fractional products of engineered cells and bacteria is a practical necessity and a pragmatic reality.

References

1. Kolff WJ. (1968) To live without heart and kidneys. *Proc Eur Dial Transplant Assoc* **1**: 21–24.
2. Friedman EA. (1976) Feasibility of a bionic kidney. *Proc Int Conf Cybernetics Soc*, pp. 189–194.
3. Jacobs C, Broyer M, Brunner FP, *et al*. (1980) Combined report on regular dialysis and transplantation in Europe, XI 1980. *Proc Eur Dial Transplant Assoc* **18**: 4–58.
4. Berlyne GM. (1982) Over 50 and uremic equals death. The failure of the British National Health Service to provide adequate dialysis facilities. *Nephron* **31**(3): 189–190.
5. Friedman EA, Delano BG. (1981) Can the world afford trauma therapy? In: *Proc 8th Int Congr Nephrol*, Athens Greece, pp. 677–683, S. Karger.
6. Friedman EA. (1995) Facing the reality: The world cannot afford uremia therapy at the start of the 21st century. *Artif Organs* **19**: 481–485.
7. U.S. Renal Data System, USRDS 2008 Annual Data Report: *Atlas of Chronic Kidney Disease and End-Stage Renal Disease in the United States*, Chap. 12, International Comparisons. National Institutes of Health, National Institute of Diabetes and Digestive and Kidney Diseases, Bethesda, MD.
8. Friedman EA. (1993) Nephrology and the rationing of health care. *Contrib Nephrol* **102**: 230–236.
9. Poikolainen K, Eskola J. (1988) Health services resources and their relation to mortality from causes amenable to health care intervention: A cross-national study. *Int J Epidemiol* **17**: 86–89.
10. Valek A, Wing AJ. (1984) Development of dialysis and transplant activity in the world during the seventies of the 20th century. *Z Exp Chir Transplant Künstliche Organe* **17**: 86–89.
11. Friedman EA. (1994) Revelations behind a fallen curtain: Dialysis restriction and the Berlin wall. *Nephrol Dial Transplant* **9**: 242–243.

12. Friedman EA. (1996) ESRD therapy: An American success story. *JAMA* **275**: 1118–1122.
13. Friedman EA, Delano BG. (1981) Can the world afford uremia therapy? *Proc 8th Internat Congr Nephrol,* Athens, pp. 677–683, S. Karger.
14. Chang TM. (2007) 50th anniversary of artificial cells: Their role in biotechnology, nanomedicine, regenerative medicine, blood substitutes, bioencapsulation, cell/stem cell therapy and nanorobotics. *Artif Cells Blood Substit Immobil Biotechnol* **35**(6): 545–554.
15. Chang TMS. (1964) Semipermeable microcapsules. *Science* **146**: 524–527.
16. Chang TM, MacIntosh FC, Mason SG. (1996) Semipermeable aqueous microcapsules. 1. Preparation and properties. *Can J Physiol Pharmacol* **44**: 115–128.
17. Safos S, Chang TM. (1995) Enzyme replacement therapy in ENU2 phenylketonuric mice using oral microencapsulated phenylalanine ammonia-lyase: A preliminary report. *Artif Cells Blood Substit Immobil Biotechnol* **23**: 681–692.
18 Liu ZC, Chang TM. (2009) Preliminary study on intrasplenic implantation of artificial cell bioencapsulated stem cells to increase the survival of 90% hepatectomized rats. *Artif Cells Blood Substit Immobil Biotechnol* **8**: 1–5.
19. Bruni S, Chang TM. (1995) Effect of donor strains and age of the recipient in the use of microencapsulated hepatocytes to control hyperbilirubinemia in the Gunn rat. *Int J Artif Organs* **18**: 332–339.
20. Friedman EA. (1996) Bowel as a kidney substitute in renal failure. *Amer J Kidney Dis* **28**: 943–950.
21. Thompson CJS. (1914) Terra Sigillata, a famous medicament of ancient times. *Trans XVII Internat Med Congr,* London **23**: 433–440.
22. Yatzidis H. (1964) Recherches sur l'épuration extra rénale à l'aide du charbon actif. *Nephron* **1**: 310–312.
23. Giordano C, Esposito R, Randazzo G, *et al.* (1972) Oxystarch as a gastrointestinal sorbent in uremia. In: Kluthe R, Berlyne G, Burton B (eds.), *Uremia,* pp. 231–239, Stuttgart, Georg Thieme Verlag.
24. Yatzidis H, Koutsicos D, Digenis P. (1979) Newer oral sorbents in uremia. *Clin Nephrol* **2**: 105–106.
25. Niwa T, Yazawa T, Ise M, Sugano M, Kodama T, Uehara Y, *et al.* (1991) Inhibitory effect of oral sorbent on accumulation of albumin-bound

inoxyl sulfate in serum of experimental uremic rats. *Nephron* **57**: 84–88.

26. Schloerb PR. (1990) Intestinal dialysis for kidney failure. Personal experience. *ASAIO Trans* **36**(1): 4–7.

27. Kolff WJ. (1947) *New Ways of Treating Uremia*, pp. 112, J. A. Churchill, London.

28. van Noordwijk. (1982) *J Early History Kampen Dialysis Transplant* **11**: 15–18.

29. Sparks RE, Mason NS, Meier PM, Samuels WE, Litt MH, Lindan O. (1972) Binders to remove uremic waste metabolites from the GI tract. *Trans Am Soc Artif Intern Organs* **18**(0): 458 64, 484.

30. Sparks RE, Mason NS, Meier PM, Litt MH, Lindan O. (1971) Removal of uremic waste metabolites from the intestinal tract by encapsulated carbon and oxidized starch. *Trans Am Soc Artif Intern Organs* **17**: 229–238.

31. Giordano C, Esposito R, Pluvio M. (1975) Oxycellulose and ammonia-treated oxystarch as insoluble polyaldehydes in uremia. *Kidney Int Suppl* **3**: 380–382.

32. Friedman EA, Fastook J, Beyer MM, Rattazzi T, Josephson AS. (1974) Potassium and nitrogen binding in the human gut by ingested oxidized starch. *Trans Amer Soc Artif Internal Organs* **20**: 33–43.

33. Giordano C, Esposito R, Demma G. (1968) The possibility of reducing the blood nitrogen level in humans by the administration of a polyaldehyde. *Bull Soc Ital Biol Sper* **44**: 2232–2234.

34. Okada K, Takahashi S. (1995) Correction by oral adsorbent of abnormal digestive tract milieu in rats with chronic renal failure. *Nephrol Dial Transplant* **10**: 671–676.

35. Miles AM, Fleishacker J, Hyppolite G, Zhao ZH, Distant D, Friedman EA. (1995) Oral sorbent (AST-120) slows uremia progression in 7/8th nephrectomized rates. (Abstract) *J Amer Soc Nephrology* **6**: 1024.

36. Savarino SJ. (2002) A legacy in 20th-century medicine: Robert Allan Phillips and the taming of cholera. *Clin Infect Dis* **35**(6): 713–720.

37. Young TK, Lee SC, Tang CK. (1979) Diarrhea therapy of uremia. *Clin Nephrol* **11**(2): 86–91.

38. Young TK, Lee SC, Tai LN. (1980) Mannitol absorption and excretion in uremic patients regularly treated with gastrointestinal perfusion. *Nephron* **25**: 112–116.

39. Korhonen M, Ahvenjarvi S, Vanhatalo A, Huhtanen P. (2002) Supplementing barley or rapeseed meal to dairy cows fed grass-red clover silage: Amino acid profile of microbial fractions. *J Anim Sci* **80**: 2188–2196.

40. Singh J, Singh AP, Peshin PK, Singh M, Sharma SK. (1983) Studies on the effects of total nephrectomy in sheep. *Can J Comp Med* **47**: 217–221.

41. Watts C, Campbell JR. (1970) Biochemical changes following bilateral nephrectomy in the bovine. *Res Vet Sci* 11508–11514.

42. Virtanen AI. (1996) Milk production of cows on protein-free feed. *Science* **53**: 1603–1614.

43. Setala K. (1984) The promise of enzymes in therapy of uremia. I. Theoretical basis-bowel physiology. *Nephron* **37**: 1–6.

44. Setälä K. (1978) Bacterial enzymes in uremia management. *Kidney Int Suppl* **8**: S194–S202.

45. Prakash S, Chang TMS. (1996) Microencapsulated genetically engineered live *E. coli* DH5 cells administered orally to maintain normal plasma urea level in uremic rats. *Nature Med* **2**: 883–887.

46. Ranganathan N, Friedman EA, Tam P, Rao V, Ranganathan P, Dheer R. (2009) Probiotic dietary supplementation in patients with stage 3 and 4 chronic kidney disease: A 6-month pilot scale trial in Canada. *Curr Med Res Opin* **25**: 1919–1930.

47. Ezendam J, van Loveren H. (2006) Probiotics: Immunomodulation and evaluation of safety and efficacy. *Nutr Rev* **641**: 1–14.

Index